NAIL STYLE

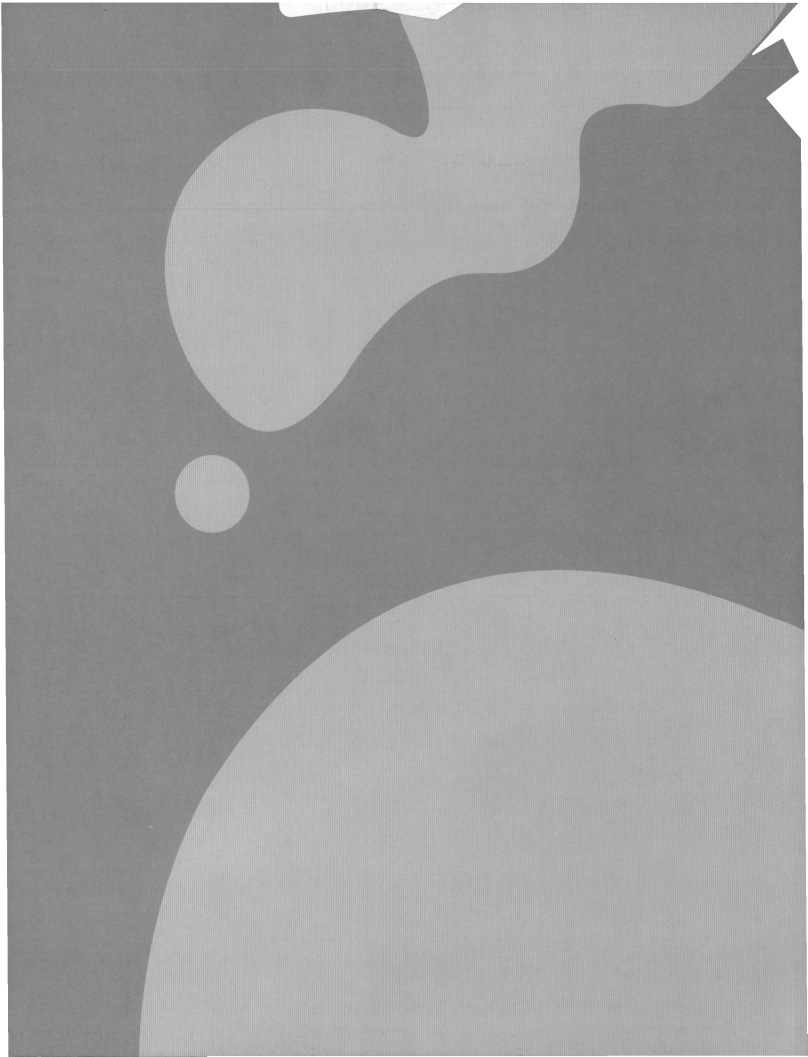

NAIL STYLE

AMAZING DESIGNS BY THE WORLD'S LEADING NAIL TECHS

Helena Biggs

ARCTURUS

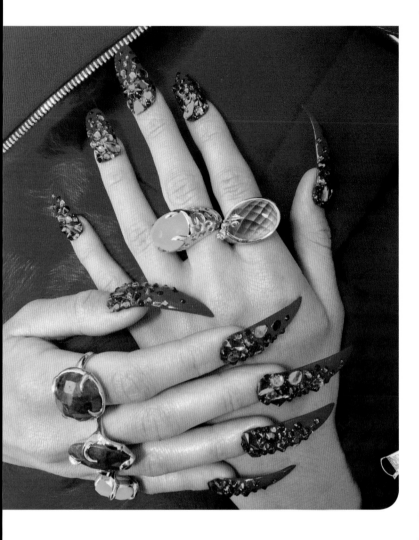

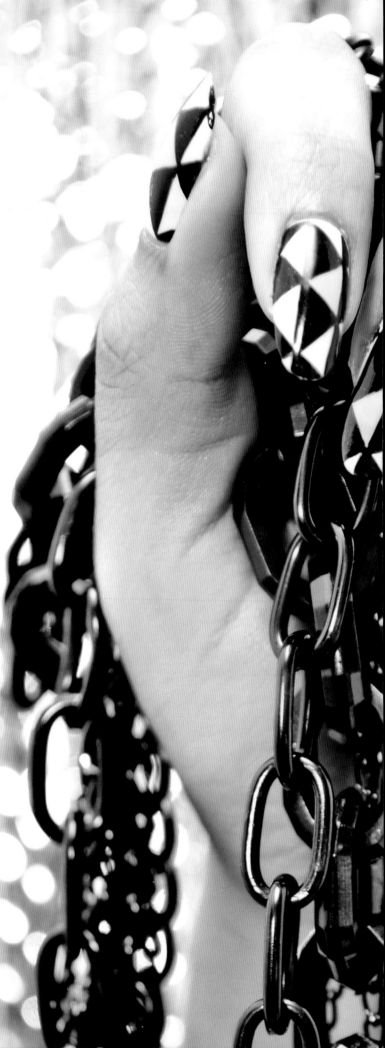

ARCTURUS

This edition published in 2014 by Arcturus Publishing Limited
26/27 Bickels Yard, 151–153 Bermondsey Street,
London SE1 3HA

Copyright © Arcturus Holdings Limited

All rights reserved. No part of this publication may be reproduced,
stored in a retrieval system, or transmitted, in any form or by
any means, electronic, mechanical, photocopying, recording or
otherwise, without written permission in accordance with the
provisions of the Copyright Act 1956 (as amended). Any person or
persons who do any unauthorised act in relation to this publication
may be liable to criminal prosecution and civil claims for damages.

ISBN: 978-1-78404-194-6
AD004208UK

Author: Helena Biggs

Printed in China

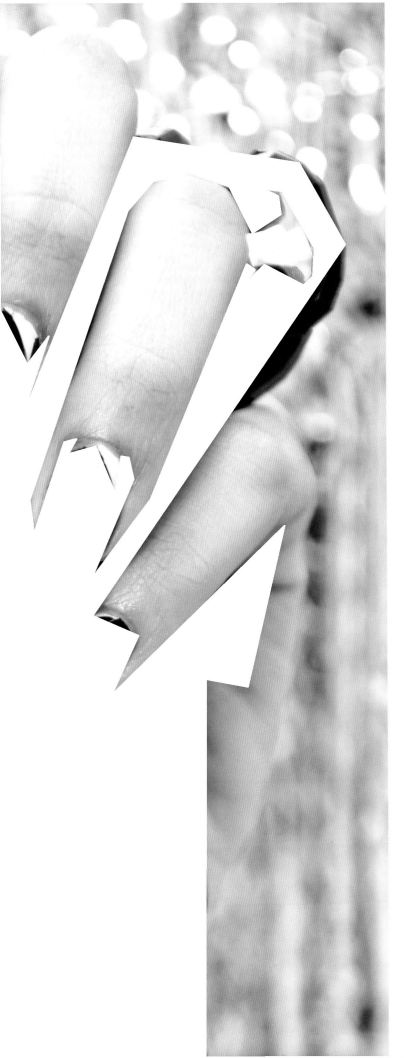

Contents

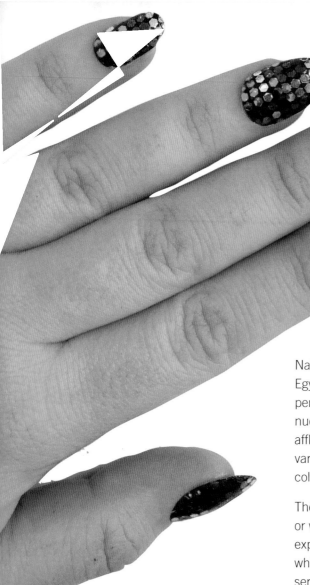

Introduction

While the word 'style' is commonly associated with fashion and trends, in reality it is influenced by numerous factors. The key to recognizing these is to understand that style is a way to express our inner thoughts, interests or values on an outer level. This is done through the way we speak, behave and dress, as well as how we wear our hair and our nails. Individual taste, lifestyle and even our surroundings can dictate our style choices. Our style is a form of self-expression – a look adopted to communicate personal tastes, a theme or a message.

Nail adornment began 5000 years ago, when henna was used on nails by the Egyptians to signify social order, and since then has developed into a signifier of personality, interests and self. Despite the available shades being limited to red and nude in the 1920s, the use of nail polish became representative of a glamorous, affluent figure. Later, the mass production of nail lacquer led to the advent of a variety of shades and paved the way to greater expression of taste through nail colour and now design, shape and texture.

The shade chosen by the wearer was once based simply on their favourite colour or whether it complemented an ensemble. Trend-followers in the Sixties began to express their appreciation for art and 'flower power' with floral designs on nails, while in the 1970s, long, stiletto nails represented affluence. As professional nail services became increasingly popular in the 1980s and 1990s, so did products such as the liquid and powder acrylic system that encouraged experimentation with nail shape and sculpture, depending on preference and practicality. Hip-hop culture saw nail design soar, as artistes in the music business expressed themselves through the designs on their sparkling talons.

With the increased social acceptability of nail design and an abundance of products for nails both in the salon and in high-street stores, the possibilities for expression are limited only by imagination and practicality. Various nail stickers, colours and decals mean that as consumers, we can experiment with a style to suit our mood, or try one that is influenced by something we admire. Our imagination and individuality are powerfully conveyed through the non-verbal message of style, and a trained nail technician or nail artist can further enhance our self-expression with professional nail products, sculpting designs that are more extravagant than those that can be achieved with nail stickers and decals.

Fashion designers recognize that to convey the inspiration behind their collections they need to combine all aspects of their models' appearance for the most powerful impact, from hair and make-up to nail art. High fashion is arguably one of the most influential factors for nail style, and its influence means that the possibility for nail designs is now infinite; with the help of professional nail technicians, almost any style can be achieved.

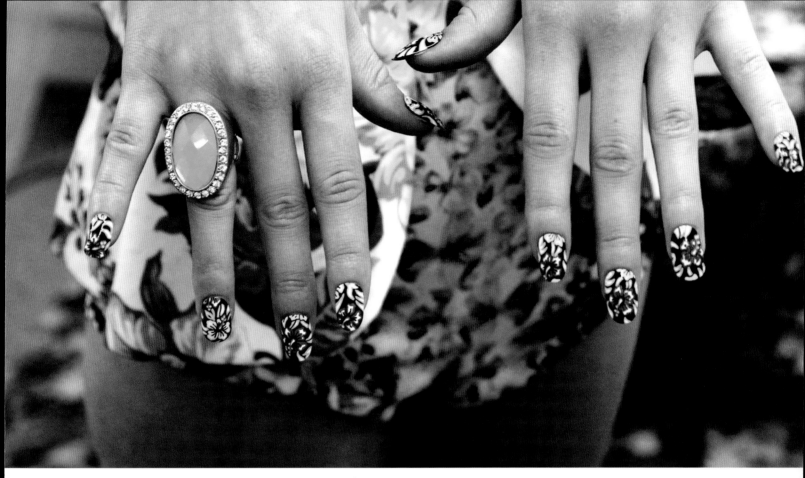

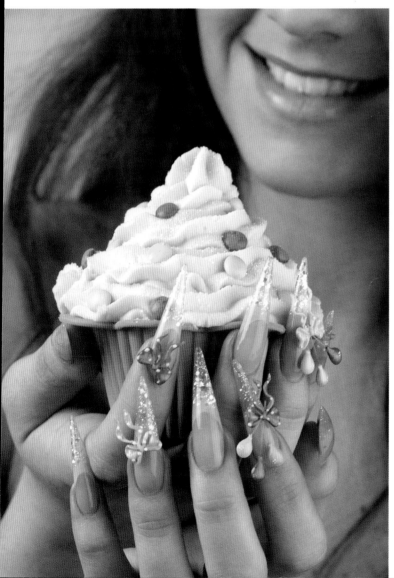

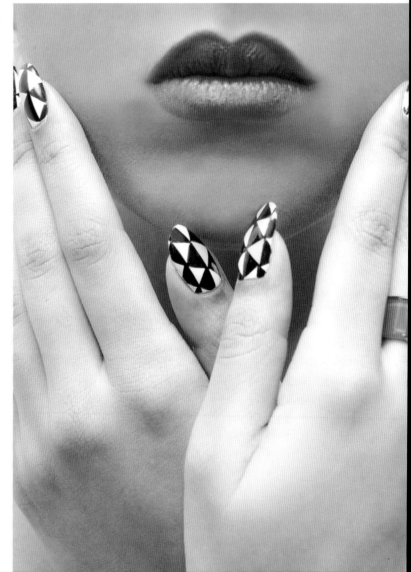

Preparation

Before commencing any nail style, it is important to prepare the nail to ensure the longevity of the look and create a smooth canvas on which to work.

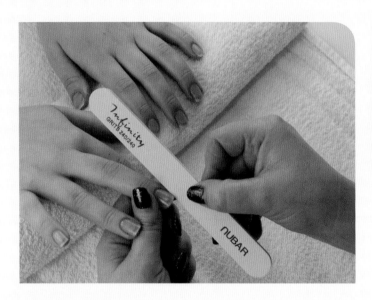

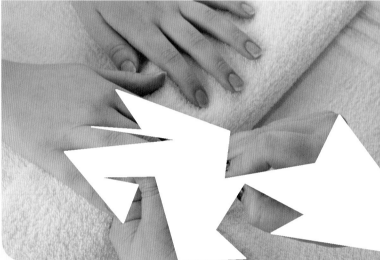

1 File the nails gently to the desired shape.

2 Tidy the cuticle area by pushing the cuticles away from the base and sidewalls of the nail, using a cuticle tool.

SHAPE AND STYLE

Top tip

If you find it difficult to paint designs on your own nails, create them on press-on nails, then simply adhere to your natural nails when the nail paint is dry.

The shape of the nail can emphasize an individual's personal sense of style or character. The almond shape oozes femininity and elongates the fingers for a elegant appearance, whereas a nail with a sharp point – while not always practical – is often suggestive of a bold, fierce persona and is suited to those with a stand-out style.

However, the shape of the nails is often dictated by practical needs, lifestyle or even age. School rules or sporting activities may call for short, square nails, and similarly some jobs, particularly in the food and healthcare sectors, may require short, well-filed nails. It's careers in these sectors that can also dictate an individual's nail style, requiring a minimal, natural nail with no nail polish or overlays.

Recommended kit

Base coat

Buffer

Cotton pads

Cuticle tool

Hand sanitizer

Nail file

Nail polish remover

Paper towels

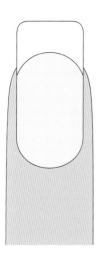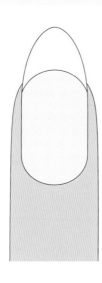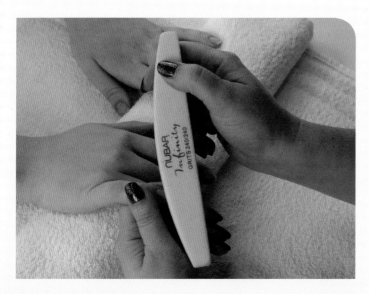

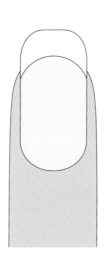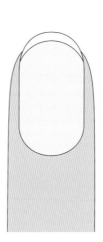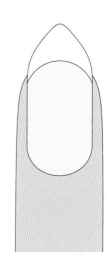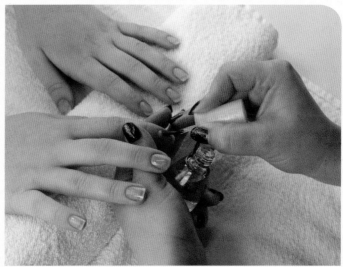

3 Use a buffer to lightly buff the nail plate and leave a smooth surface for application.

4 Apply a thin layer of base coat, leaving a 1 mm gap around the edge of the nail. Allow to dry before beginning your nail design.

Square nails *Classic and timeless, these are ideal for balancing out narrow, long fingers.*

Oval nails *These suit everyone and give the illusion of an elongated nail bed.*

Squoval nails *Softer-looking than a square nail, they still maintain the same qualities.*

Round nails *Less prone to breakage, round nails also soften larger hands or fingers.*

Pointed nails *A fashion-forward style that elongates the hand and fingers.*

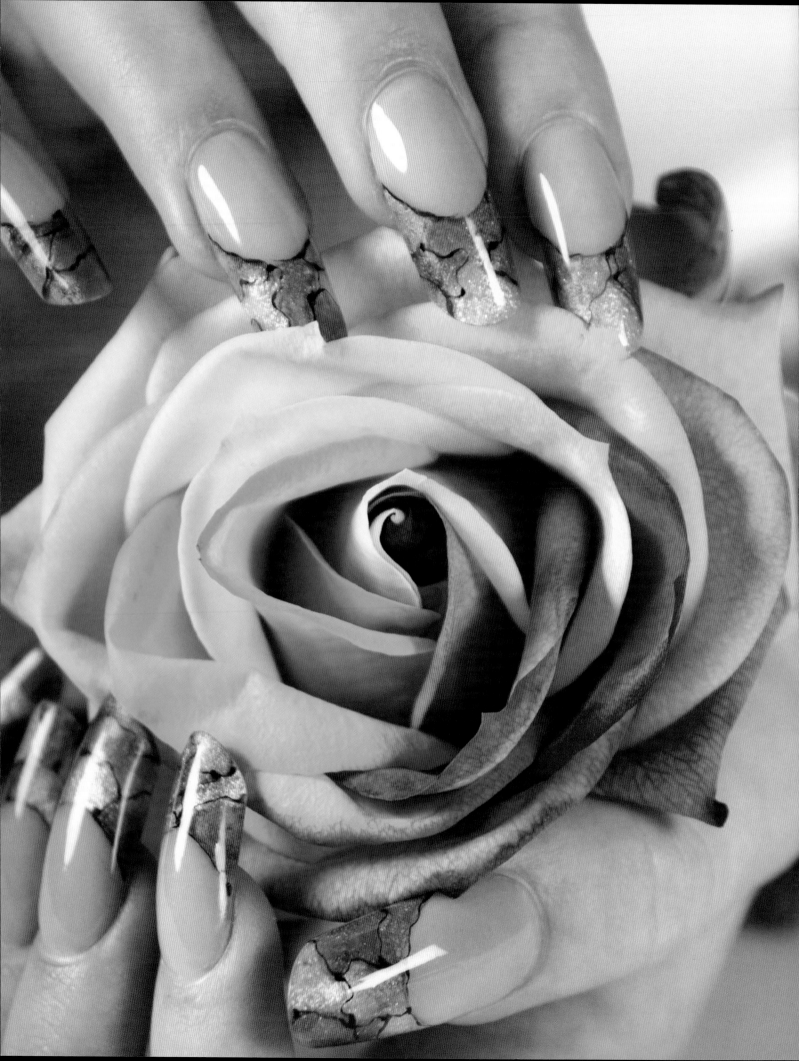

CHAPTER ONE

THE WORLD AROUND US

Natural and urban scenes offer plenty of inspiration for nail styling. The varied colours, textures and patterns of our surroundings can serve to influence the artistry used in nail design, with the design showing an appreciation of the natural world or interest in unique forms.

Landscapes are detailed and intriguing and when translated onto nails, they can show patriotism or an appreciation of the particular geography of the land. Animal prints are a popular nail style as they are relatively easy to create, yet offer an eye-catching look. You can replicate the coats of zebras, leopards and snakes with dotting tools and nail stripers, or look to birds, flora and marine life for colour inspiration.

For additional creativity, use the influence of your surroundings to add texture to nail designs. Consider sticking artificial feathers onto nails if you find hand-painted design tricky, or stick dried flowers onto pre-painted nails with glue before sealing with a topcoat to take some of the difficulty out of nail artistry.

Left *French-style nails with a multi-coloured, marbled-effect tip by Gemma Lambert.*

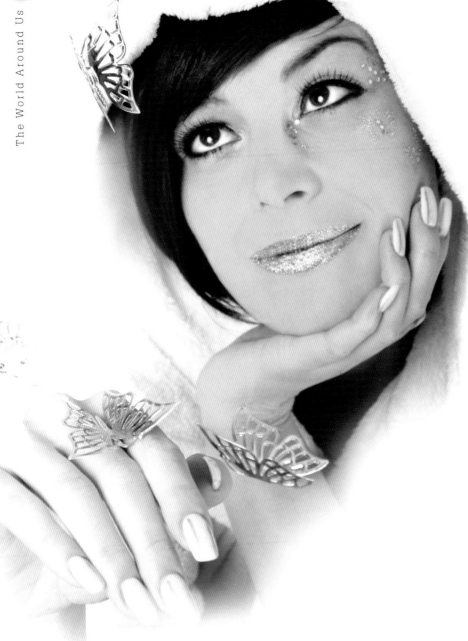

Seasons and Elements

Seasons dictate trends in the commercial nail colour world, as they do for fashion choices and the colours and practicalities of clothing collections. Darker shades and glitters are often prevalent in the winter months, with pastels in the spring and bright shades in the summer to complement the natural colours and holidays relevant to the season.

Complement the seasons with nail shades that pay homage to each. Consider drawing inspiration from the elements earth, water, wind and fire for designs to suit your personality and use nail decals and art products to bring the nail style to life.

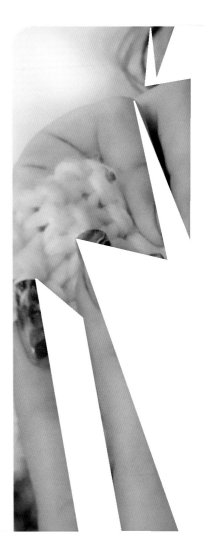

Above *Wintry white nails with silver detailing by Sam Biddle.*

Left *Stiletto-shaped nails featuring shades of white, pale blue and silver, inspired by an ice queen theme by Gemma Lambert.*

Right *Autumn-themed nails by Gemma Lambert with hand-painted detailing and a 3D, sculpted leaf design on feature nails.*

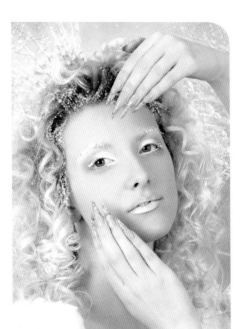

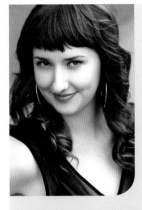

TECHNICIAN PROFILE
Fleury Rose, USA

Born in Connecticut, USA, Fleury Rose has always had a passion for painting, drawing and illustration. She graduated with a degree in Fine Art in 2009, having developed a love for watercolours, oil painting and ink drawing. She resides in Brooklyn, New York, where she pursues her creativity.

Inspired by Japanese nail art magazines and eager to paint on small canvases, Fleury founded a nail blog, Fleuryrosenails, to showcase her designs. The interest in her work became overwhelming and she had so many requests to do people's nails that she began to build her nail empire, working in a salon by appointment only and creating designs for a number of magazines and blogs, including *Teen Vogue* and *Paper* magazines.

Fleury is US Nail Ambassador for cult British beauty brand Illamasqua and is recognized for her bold take on nail art.

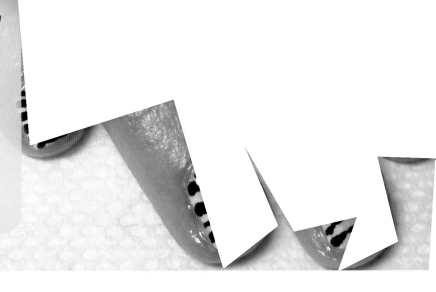

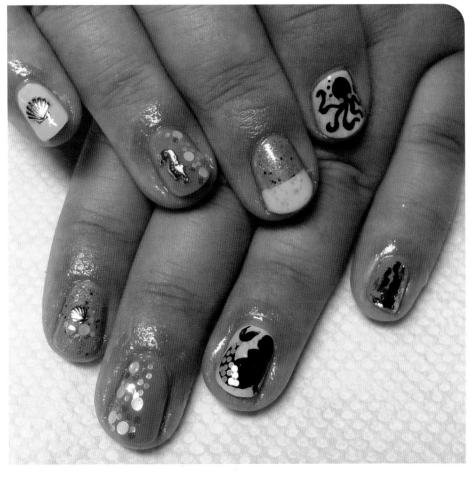

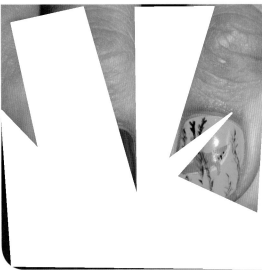

Left *Hand-painted sea-themed nails featuring glitter and embellishments.*

Top *Nails inspired by tiger prints, with hand-painted stripes on an ombre-effect base.*

Above *Shark nail art designs hand-painted onto an opaque nail base.*

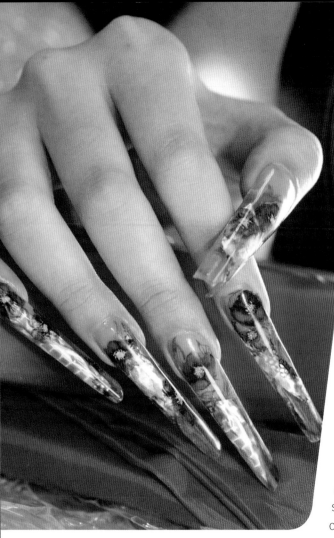

The Garden of Life

Plants and flowers are commonly used in nail design, as their beauty and colour afford a wealth of design opportunity for all skill levels. Stencils and stickers offer an easy, speedy way for floral nails or, for a unique style, consider a hand-painted design using brushes and stripers.

Aesthetically, flowers are pleasing to the eye and are suggestive of femininity. As they're also incredibly variable in appearance, they can suit all personalities; use bright colours and basic flower designs on short nails for a fun, fresh look – perfect for a festival or summer event – or consider getting a technician to sculpt flowers onto an extended nail for a glamorous, elegant style. A floral nail design can be worn in a subtle manner, with just one or two flowers on an accent nail, or all over, in a big, blooming design, dependent on the wearer's taste.

As well as flowers, elegant creatures such as swans can offer intriguing nail styles, or look to other birds and insects such as butterflies for alternative colour and design inspiration.

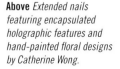

Above *Extended nails featuring encapsulated holographic features and hand-painted floral designs by Catherine Wong.*

Right *A beautiful butterfly-themed set of nails by Catherine Wong, comprising multi-coloured nail extensions and 3D butterflies crafted using professional nail products.*

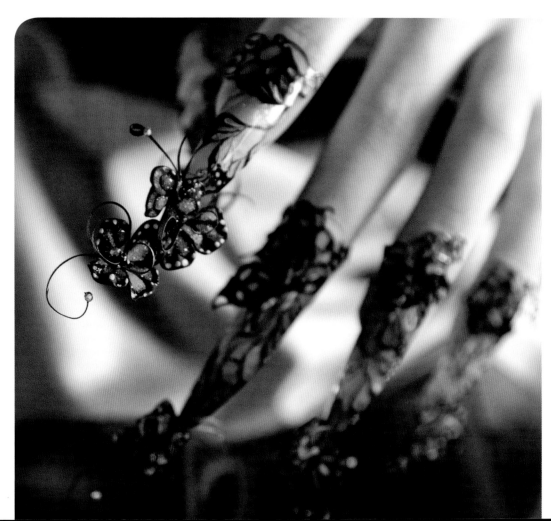

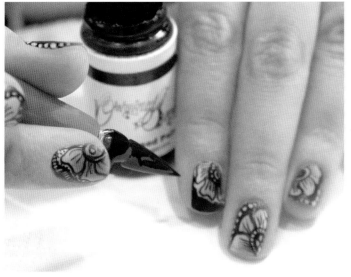

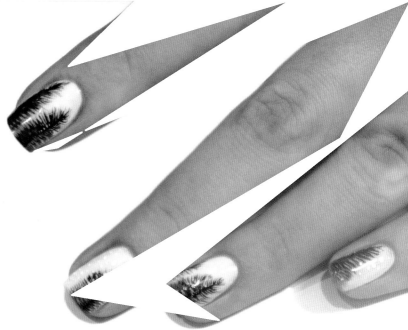

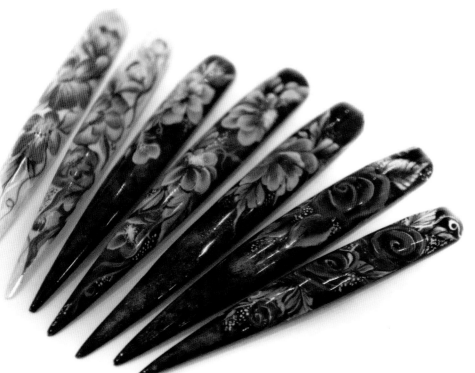

Left *Nail tips with an assortment of floral designs created by Sam Biddle.*

Top left *Colourful ombre nails with large floral nail art created by Sam Biddle using a nail art pen.*

Above *White nails with hand-painted tree designs and a sprinkling of glitter by Sam Biddle.*

Below left *A French manicure with floral details on the ring fingers created using the one-stroke nail art method by Eva Darabos.*

Below right *French-style nails in a square shape with lilac flower detailing by Eva Darabos.*

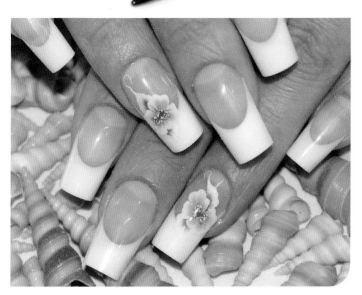

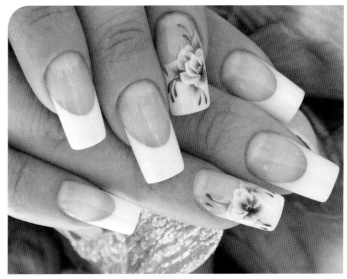

PROJECT: FLORAL NAILS by Gemma Lambert

**Gemma Lambert shows how to jazz up plain, polished nails
with a fancy hand-painted floral design.**

You will need

1 Two thin nail brushes

2 Base coat

3 Three coloured nail polishes

4 One white nail polish

5 Top coat

6 Crystals or diamantés

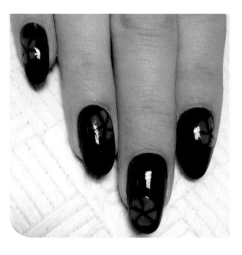

1 Apply base coat and two coats of your chosen shade of nail polish. Allow to dry.

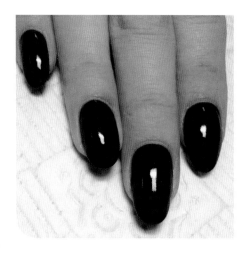

2 Using a thin brush and a lighter nail-polish shade, create five triangular shapes on each nail to form the petals. Leave space in between each shape and alter the position of the design on each nail.

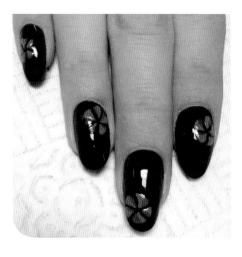

3 When the petals are dry, take a contrasting shade and paint over half of each petal.

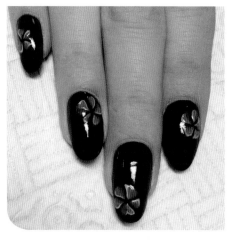

4 Using a fine brush dipped in white nail polish, add an accent to each of the petals, along half of the top edge and down the side of each.

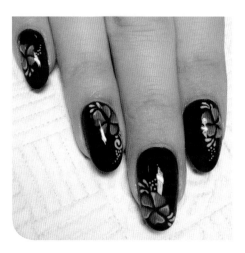

5 Continuing with the white shade, enhance your design with leaf-effects each side and add some small dots in a cluster. Allow to dry thoroughly then apply top coat. While this is still wet, add a diamanté or crystal to the centre of each flower.

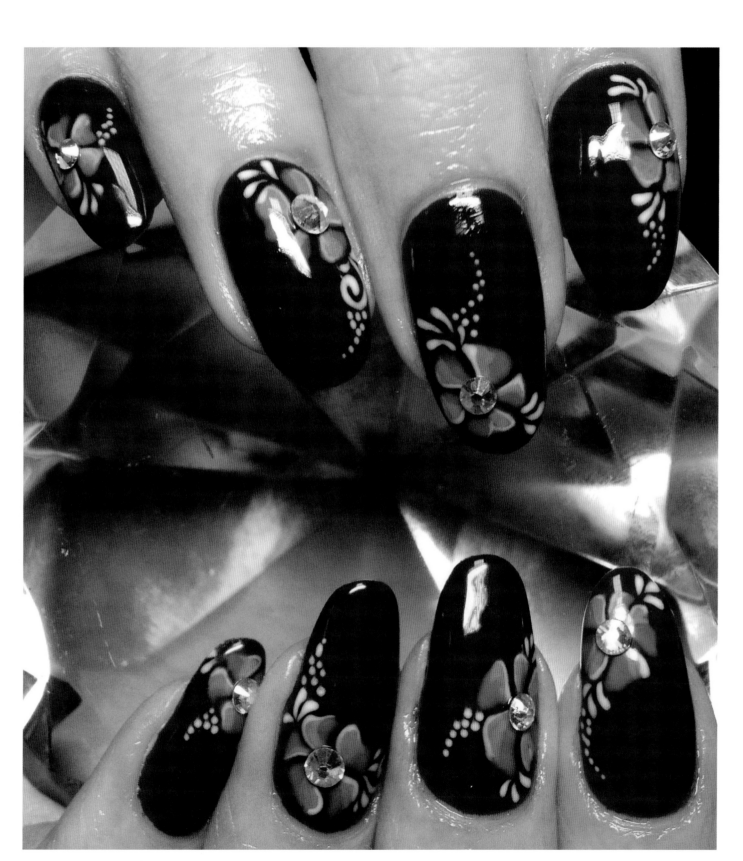

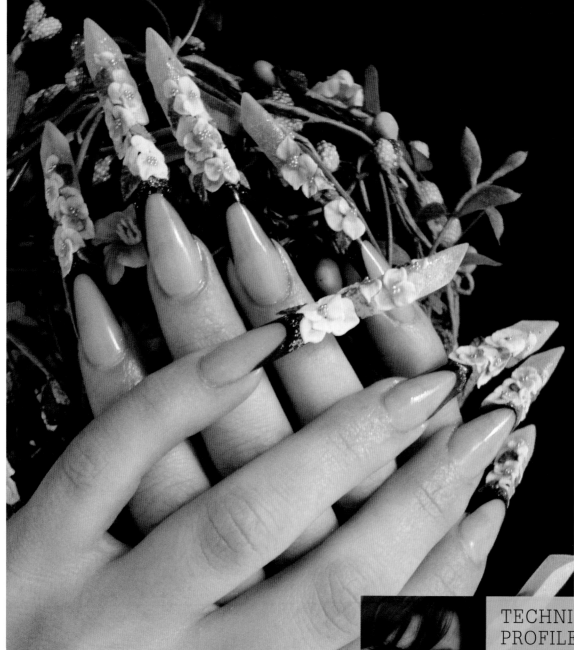

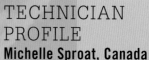

Left *Nails sculpted to a 'lipstick' shape and finished with 3D floral designs and embellishments.*

Right *Stiletto-shaped nails in autumnal shades with floral embellishments.*

Below left *Enhanced nails with flowers created using professional nail products and featuring diamanté detailing and a touch of sparkle.*

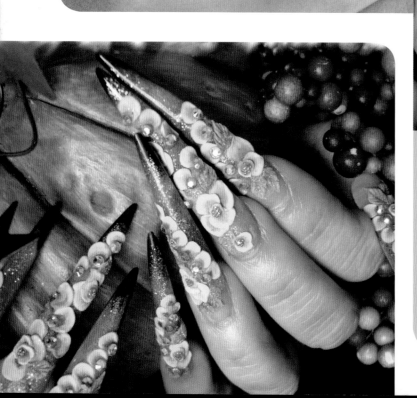

TECHNICIAN PROFILE
Michelle Sproat, Canada

Michelle has been in the beauty industry for more than 30 years. Devoted to the development of new and existing nail talent, she travels the world to share her passion for new and existing nail techniques as well as running her nail salon in Ontario. A seasoned nail competitor and champion, Michelle has a passion for new and exciting nail techniques which ensures that her nail artistry is always cutting edge. She worked for renowned nail brand OPI as a trainer and international nail artist for more than two decades, judging competitions and giving presentations all over the world. Michelle's work has featured in a number of consumer and nail trade magazines and she now works as a distributor of Odyssey Nail Systems products, sharing her design skills and application tips with fellow nail technicians.

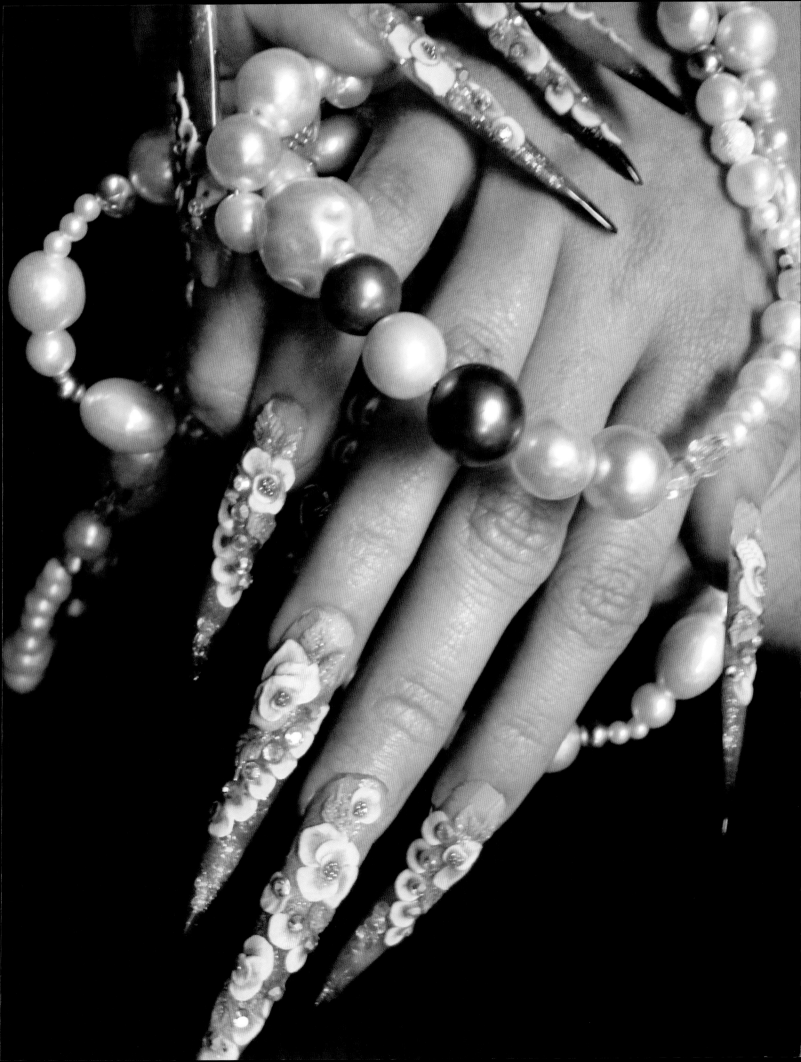

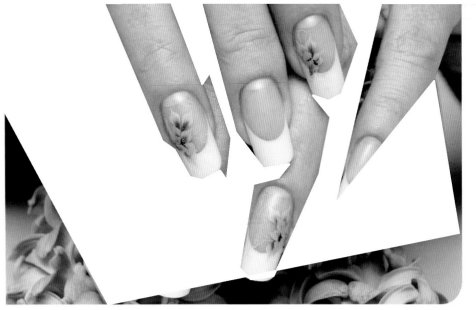

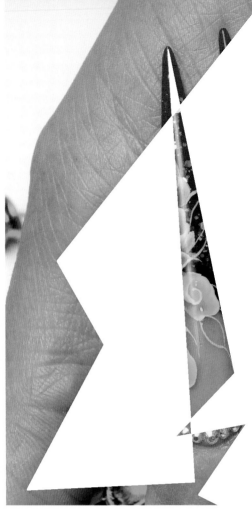

Above *French nails with a rounded tip by Eva Darabos, with hand-painted detailing on feature nails inspired by real flowers.*

Left *Striking blue stiletto nails by Eva Darabos with diamanté embellishments at the cuticle and floral detailing.*

Right *Eye-catching stiletto-shaped nails by Eva Darabos with a red glitter tip, embellishments by the cuticle and floral nail art created using the one-stroke art technique.*

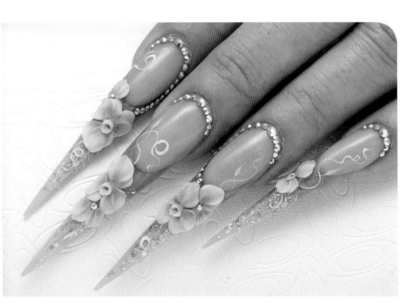

Image Gallery

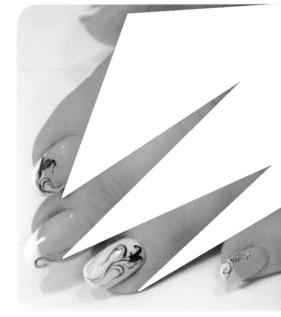

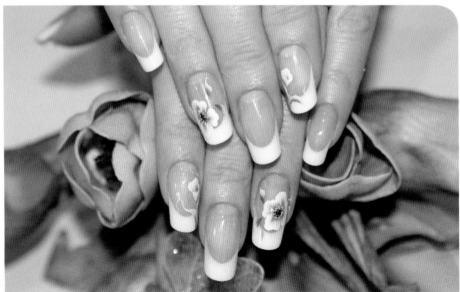

Above *Tulip-inspired artistry on a French manicure base and block-colour ring finger by Sam Biddle.*

Left *Pretty French manicure-style nails with delicate floral detailing on feature nails by Eva Darabos.*

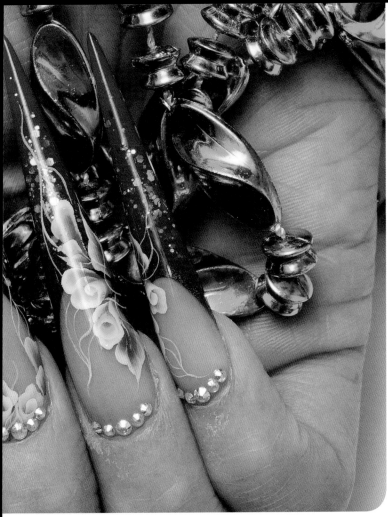

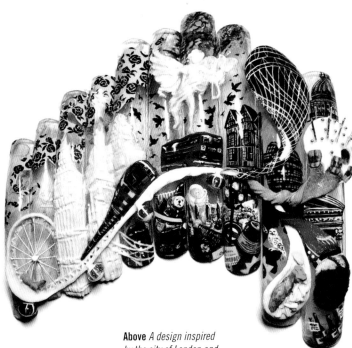

Above *A design inspired by the city of London and created on false nail tips by Megumi Mizuno, using both nail paints and professional nail products.*

Below *Peacock-inspired nails in a stiletto shape by Sam Biddle.*

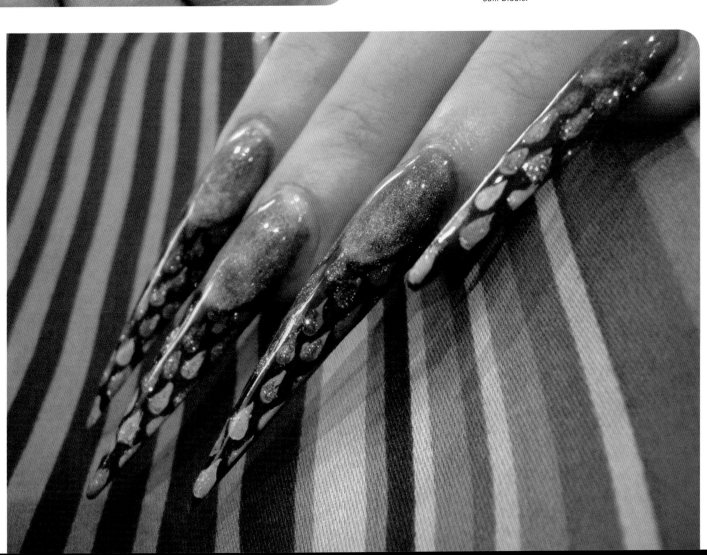

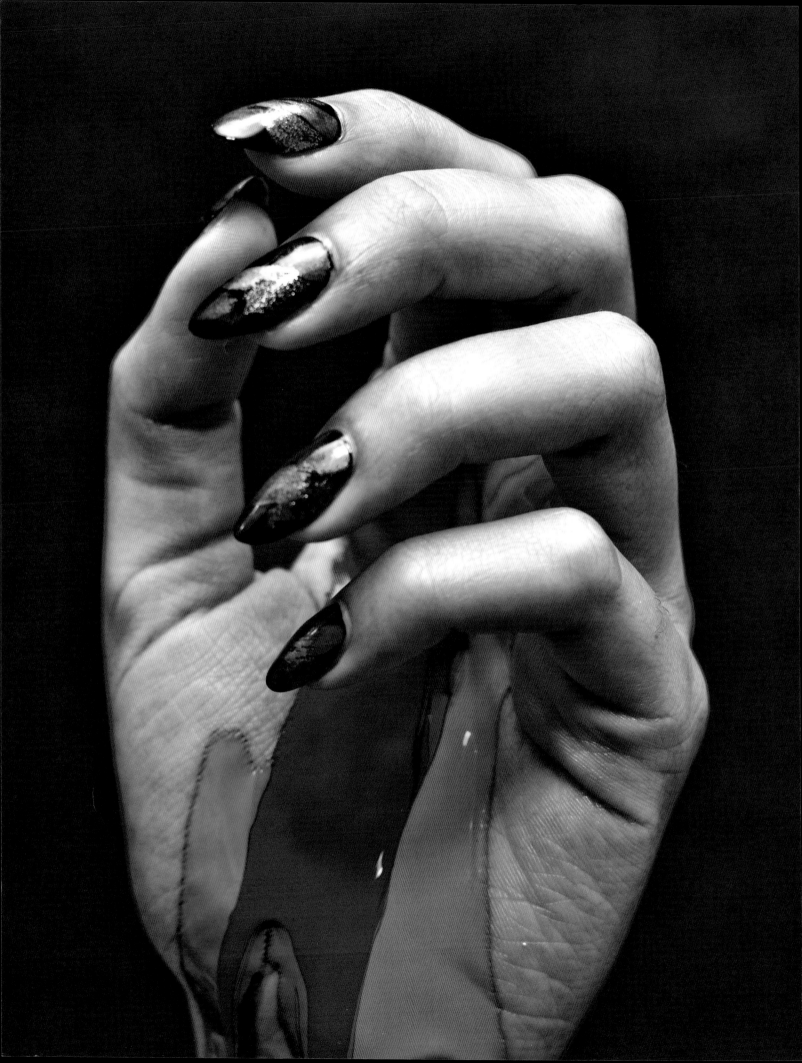

CHAPTER TWO

ART

Art is so diverse in form and subjective in matter that it presents an endless amount of inspiration for nail styles. A key form of expression, artworks unveil thoughts, desires and passions for settings and specific characters which can then be translated into nail design.

Whichever style of art you are attracted to, whether it be Impressionism, Pop Art or Cubism, for example, you can take elements of a design and create your own interpretation or try to replicate the design whole – or even opt for a freestyle design based on your own mood or feeling.

Those with a desire for subtle nail art may choose to look to the works of Monet or Cézanne, using soft shades and free brushstrokes. This kind of style is ideal for those who have a love of art but an unsteady hand for design. Alternatively, you can use stencils for Banksy-style designs and thin tape to echo elements of structural art and create clean, straight lines.

If you are confident with nail polishes, paints and thin brushes, consider portrait work or detailed replicas – perhaps the iconic *Mona Lisa* or, for a religious homage, *The Last Supper*. At the opposite extreme, for a quick-fix way to express artistic desire on nails, try to find custom nail wraps or stickers in your chosen design.

Left *A colourful design on almond-shaped nails by Ami Vega, inspired by dripping paint.*

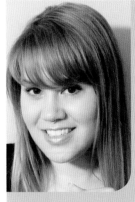

TECHNICIAN PROFILE
Astrowifey, USA

Freelance manicurist AstroWifey, aka Ashley Crowe, is passionate about nail care and design and has been immersed in the nail industry since 2008. From a background in art, she began creating designs on her own nails that attracted so much attention she trained as a manicurist in order to begin working on others.

AstroWifey builds her brand at events, private parties and photo shoots and has her own line of merchandise. Inspired by the health of natural nails, she takes pride in producing nail designs that are customized specifically for clients, taking her art background onto the canvas of the nail plate.

Creator of the first American nail art lifestyle magazine, *Tipsy Zine*, AstroWifey is listed on popular fashion and style website Refinery29 as 'Chicago's most mandatory nail artist'. She has also had her work published in *Scratch*, a leading magazine for nail professionals, and works on a freelance basis as a nail artist.

'I always encourage clients to bring their own ideas to the manicure table, whether it's a picture, an idea or theme, colour suggestions or even an item they would like to match. This gives me an idea of the client's style.' AstroWifey

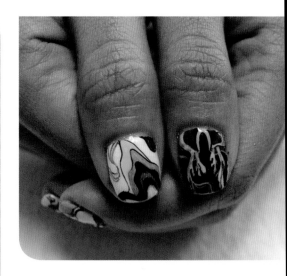

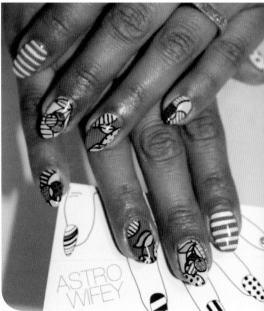

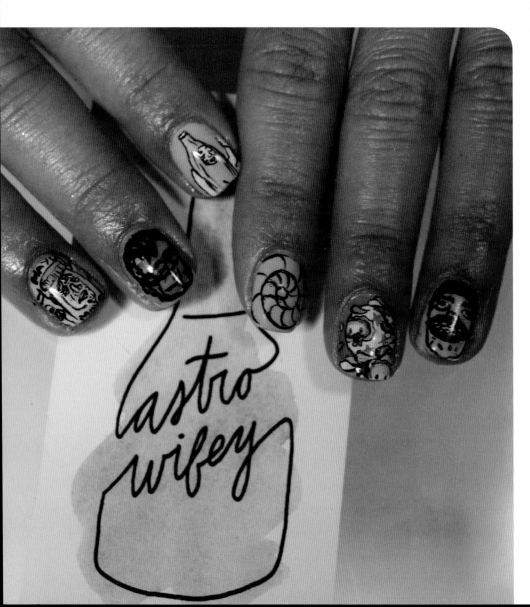

Top *An artistic freehand design using a variety of nail polish shades.*

Above *A pretty nail design in punchy shades of pink, aqua, yellow and green.*

Left *A random and imaginative hand-painted nail design, using an assortment of nail-polish shades.*

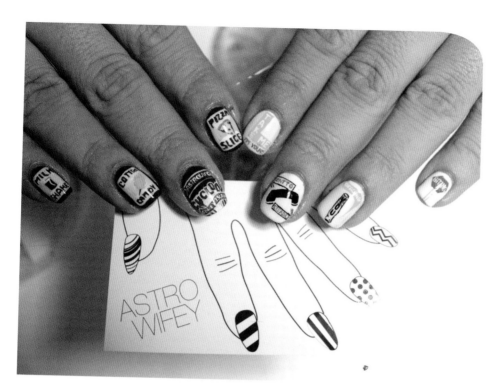

Left *Fun hand painted nail designs featuring food signs and slogans.*

Below *A random freehand nail design using an assortment of shades and varied brushstrokes, featuring gold embellishments.*

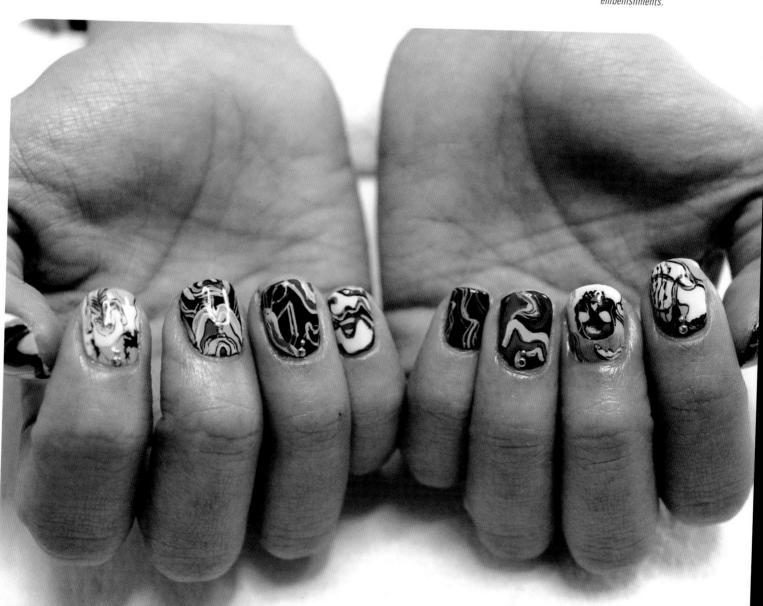

Activism and Expression Through Art

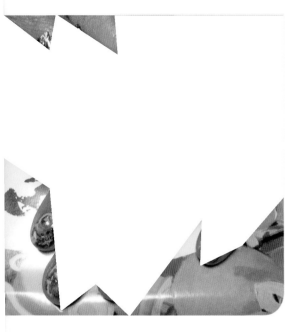

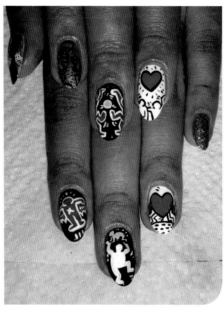

Using art as a medium for social and political expression became a feature of the 1960s, when a response to mass culture and dominant ideologies in post-war London and New York led to the Pop Art movement. Influences from popular culture saw the rise of colourful, expressive artistry mimicking the style of advertisements, commenting on the depersonalization of society by the mass media.

Through their work, Pop Artists showed that mass culture is an unavoidable entity that changes perceptions and values. Andy Warhol and Roy Lichtenstein were key figures of the movement, and a number of their designs – such as Warhol's series on Marilyn Monroe and Lichenstein's *Ten Dollar Bill* – used the duplication technique to show an increasing lack of individuality and general anonymity in society. Comic and cartoon-style works offered an ironic outlet through which to express social and political anxiety.

Two decades later, American artist Keith Haring – a friend of Andy Warhol – created works inspired by New York City street culture and the burgeoning graffiti art scene, using bright colour, bold outlines and active figures to carry socio-political themes, such as birth, death, sexuality, war and drug use. Figures of animals and humans were largely used in his works to represent various aspects of culture and convey a particular characteristic or message.

When the style of the works from these movements is adapted for nail art, the suggestion is that the wearer has an appreciation of their values. For those less inclined to express socio-political views through their nails, elements of art can be translated onto nails in a more light-hearted way, to voice beliefs, feelings and catchphrases.

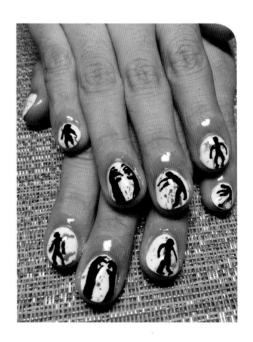

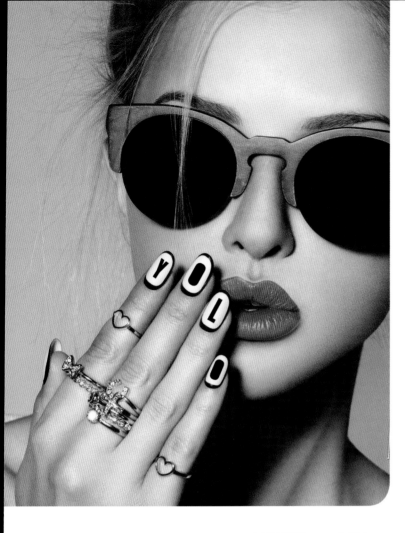

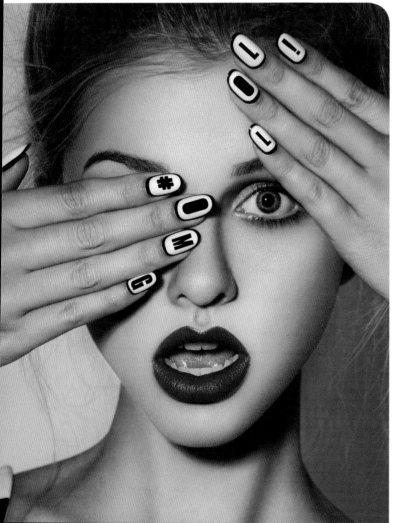

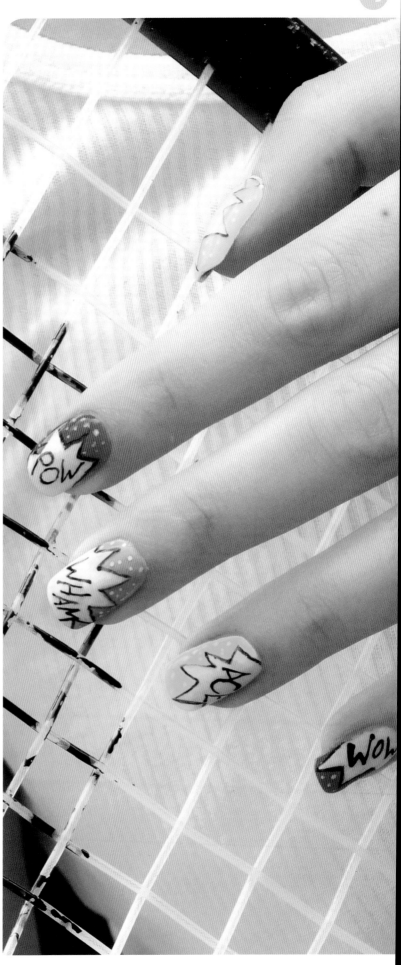

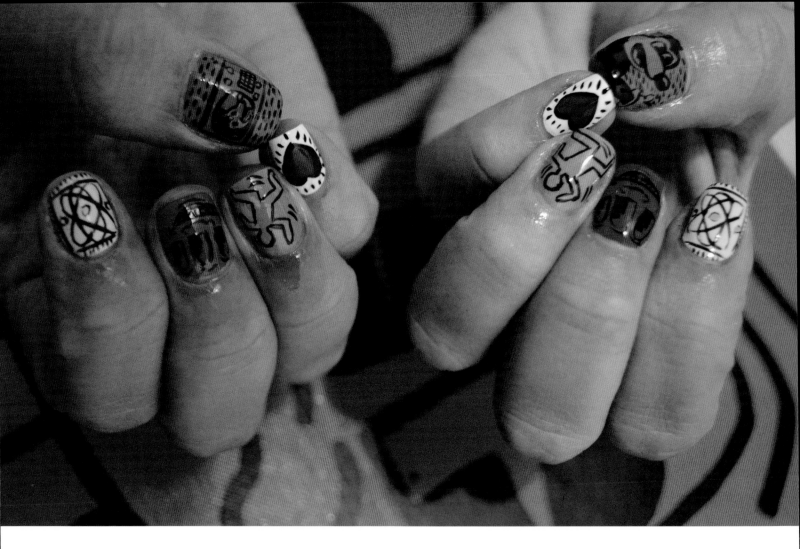

Above *A colourful nail design by Ami Vega, featuring silhouettes and hearts inspired by the artworks of Keith Haring.*

Right *Ombre-effect nails with striking white freehand nail-art effects.*

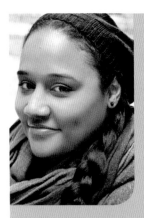

TECHNICIAN PROFILE
Ami Vega, USA

Travelling nail artist Ami Vega had her first brush with nail art at a young age, when she and a friend experimented with different polish colours on their nails. With an enthusiasm for art of all sorts, Ami started to elaborate on her nail décor and is now a highly sought-after nail artist in New York City. She seeks inspiration from Pop Art culture, bold patterns, textiles and fashion for her striking designs and chronicles her work and nail art journey on her website, elsalonsito.com.

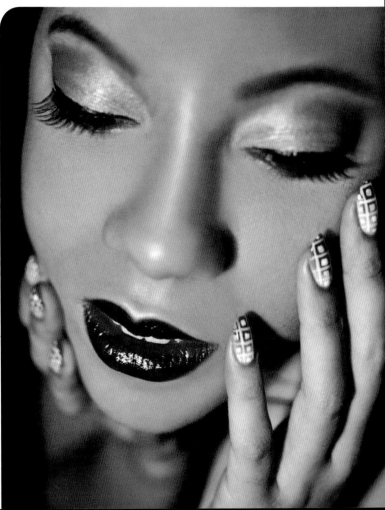

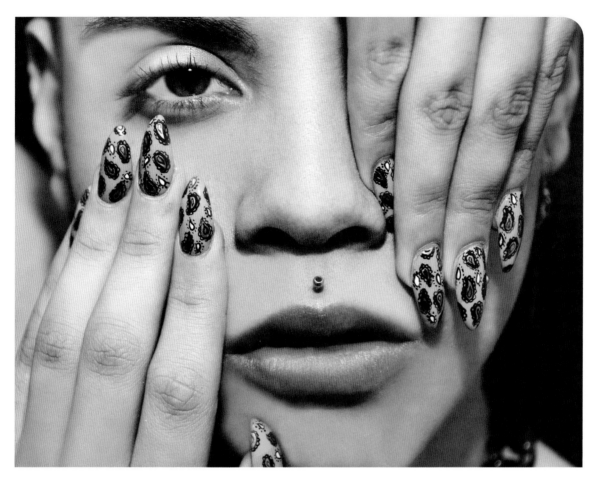

Left *A hand-painted paisley design on a colourful background.*

Below left *Pretty pastel summer-themed nails.*

Below *An alternative take on the French nail design, featuring a monochrome design on the nail tip.*

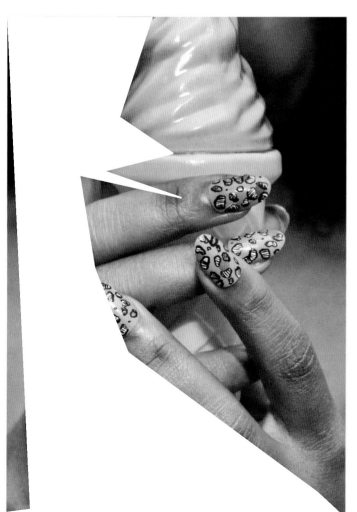

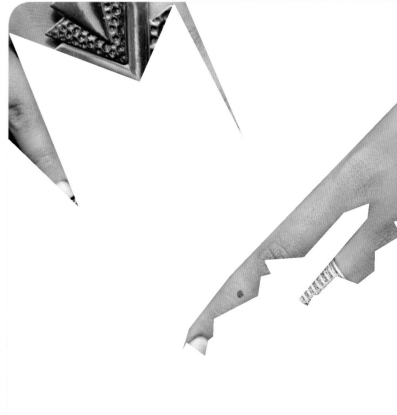

PROJECT: COLOUR-BLOCK NAILS by Ami Vega

Reflecting one of the styles associated with the Pop Art movement – image duplication to show a lack of individuality – Ami Vega creates a design using bright colours derived from 1960s art. Follow the steps below to create your own Pop Art-style nails.

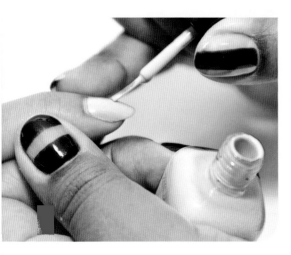

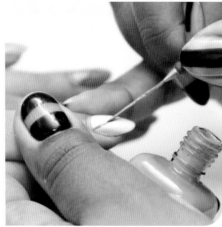

You will need

1 Thin nail brush

2 Base coat

3 Five pastel nail shades

4 Five darker nail shades

5 Top coat

1 Apply a thin layer of base coat to all nails. Apply two coats of pastel colour, using a different shade for each nail.

2 Using a darker shade of each pastel colour, use a nail-art brush to paint a diagonal line from the cuticle to the free edge of the nail.

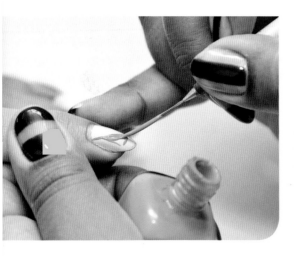

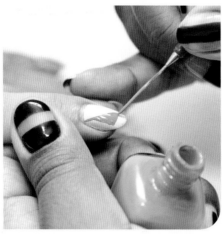

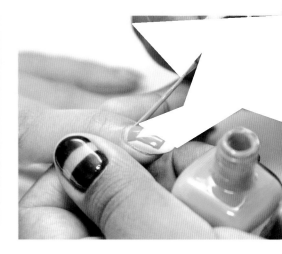

3 Outline the bottom part of the rectangle, under the diagonal line. Repeat on all nails using the relevant colour.

4 Fill in the bottom half of the rectangle that you have outlined.

5 Create the top half of the rectangle on the other side of the diagonal line. This time, fill in the outer space of the shape. Allow to dry and then apply a thin layer of top coat.

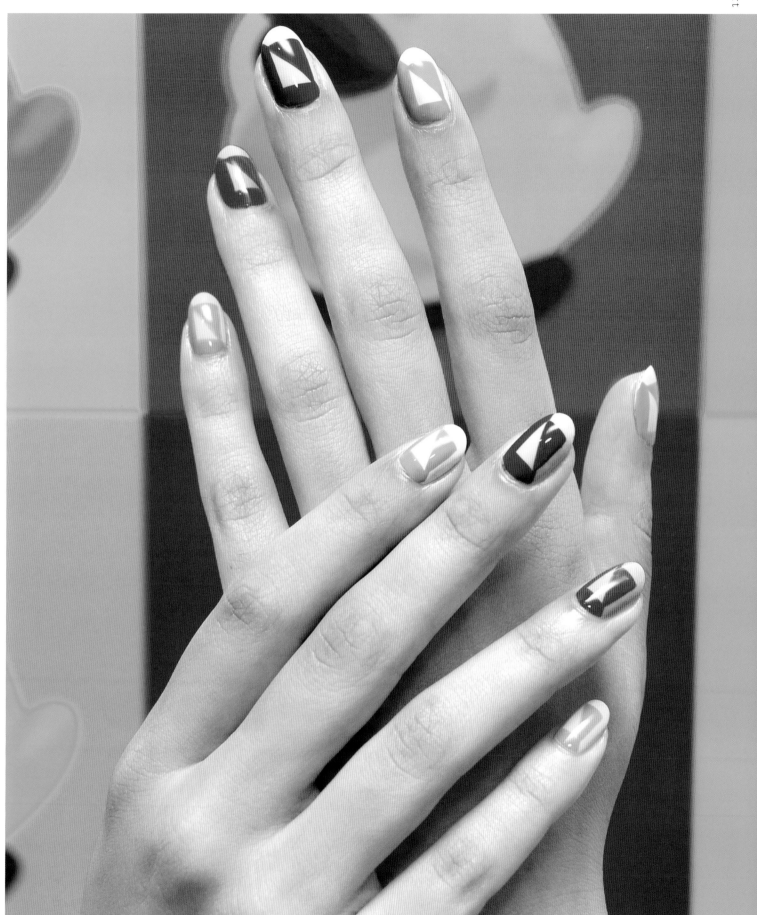

Freestyle Nail Art

A creative individual's imagination is often frenzied with colour and design ideas, with a desire to express a personal artistic style. While much of this may come from imagination and translate fluidly onto the nail canvas, some creatives may seek ideas not just from famous sculptures and canvas works, but other types of art such as cartoons and lyrics.

Freestyle nail works can be constructed using any tools the artist desires – nail stripers, polishes and brushes or stencils – in order to convey the message or design.

Right *A bold nail design inspired by the Dutch abstract artist Mondrian, created by Fleury Rose.*

Below *An expressive, striking nail-art design created by Fleury Rose, using bold shades and intense outlines.*

Below right *Watercolour-effect nails in varying shades of blue with 3D embellishments, by Fleury Rose.*

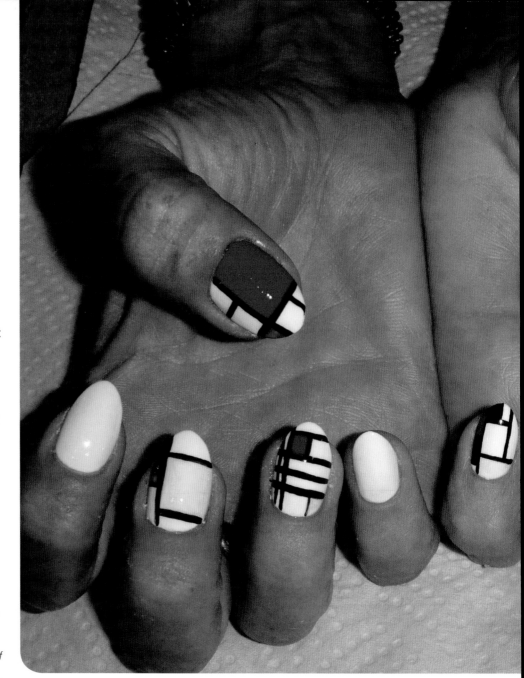

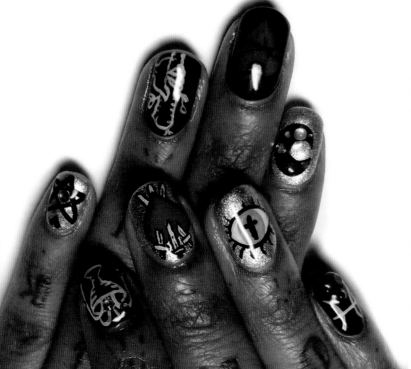

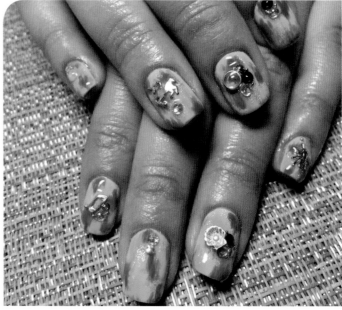

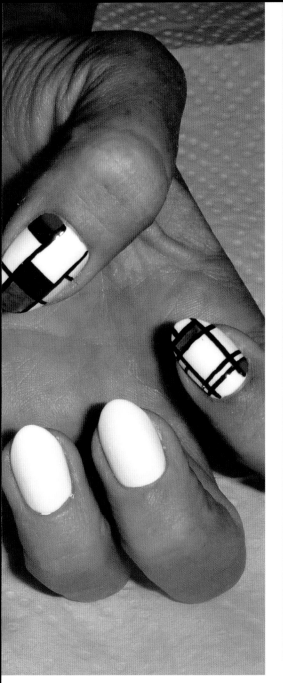

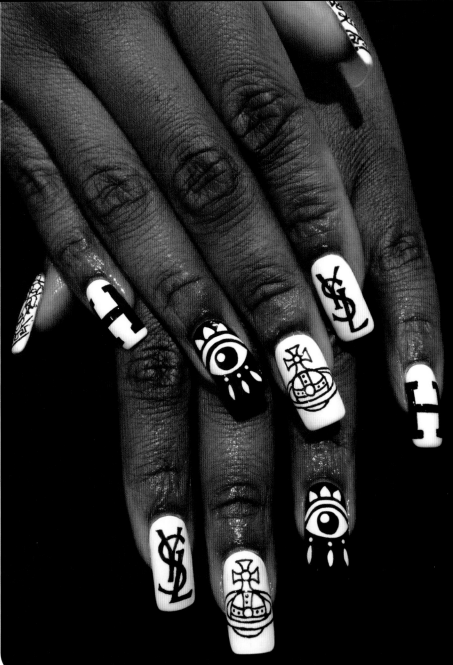

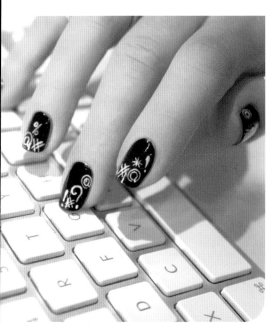

Above *Hand-painted monochrome nails that pay homage to fashion, featuring designer logos by Sophie-Harris Greenslade.*

Left *An expressive design on natural nails painted with black nail polish by Sam Biddle.*

Right *Freehand Disney-themed nail art by Megumi Mizuno, created on a white opaque nail lacquer base.*

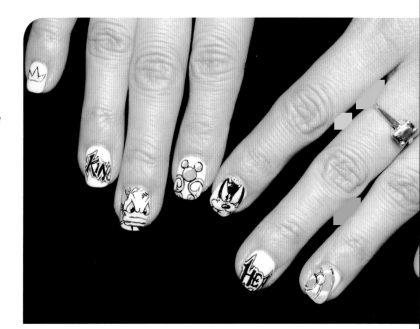

Body Art to Nail Art

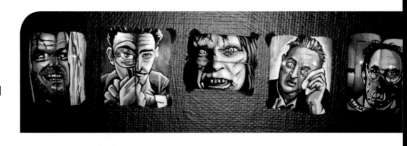

Body art is itself a form of self-decoration and self-expression, with significance to the wearer who has made the life-long commitment to showcase designs on their body. The beauty of nail design is that it requires no long-term commitment; if it is a professional enhancement it will last around three weeks, and nail polish can be changed as often as desired.

Body art and nail art can serve to complement one another, with nail art being an extension of a design. For those without body art, nail art can be a way to express their love of an image or tattoo style on a short-term basis.

Traditional tattoo style uses one part black ink, one part colour and one part skin, with thick lines. Newer styles focus on freestyling, with the wearer placing their trust in the artist to create a design with unique patterns and ideas and plenty of colour. The characteristics of both styles can be replicated on nails with polishes, paints and varied brushes.

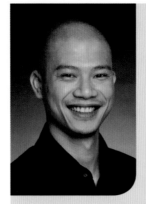

TECHNICIAN PROFILE
Vu Nguyen, USA

A graduate of the prestigious California Institute of the Arts, Vu Nguyen was an accomplished tattoo artist before he turned to nails in 2002, when his mother encouraged him to attend beauty school with her. Since graduating, he has won many nail-art competitions and is famed for incredibly detailed, hand-painted nail-art designs. Vu's work has appeared on the cover of a number of trade magazines and he has published four books on nail art.

Vu travels the world as a guest artist for nail brand OPI, training fellow nail technicians while still finding time to tattoo. He has even taught his younger brother, Robert, who is a successful nail artist in his own right, and joins forces with Vu to form OPI's A-Team, appearing at trade exhibitions and training centres worldwide.

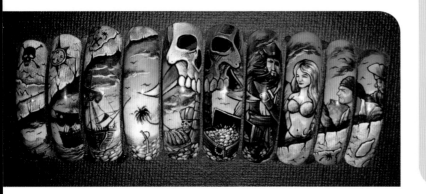

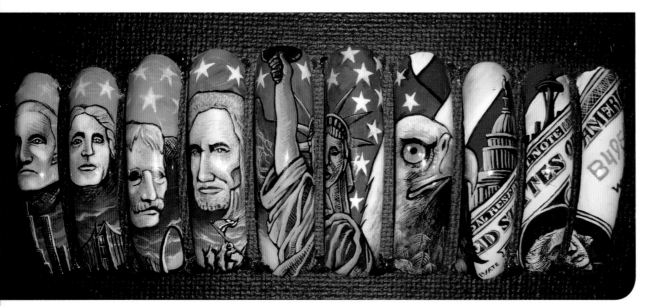

Top *Portraits of iconic film characters hand-painted onto nail tips by Vu Nguyen.*

Above left *Hand-painted nail art on nail tips by Vu Nguyen depicting a treasure island theme.*

Left
A colourful hand-painted nail design featuring iconic scenes and artefacts from the USA, created by Vu Nguyen on nail tips.

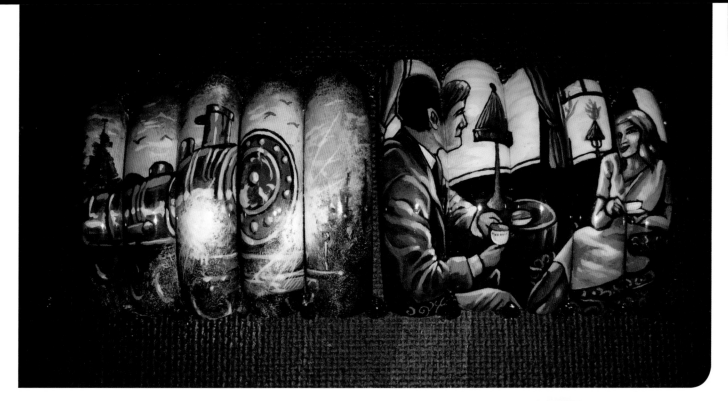

Above *A train scene by Vu Nguyen, hand-painted onto nail tips.*

Vu creates a full skull design on a matte black nail base using a nail art brush; applying two layers of white polish to the left of the skull and one to the right to create a shaded effect. He then uses a thin brush to outline the nose and create a cracked effect on the skull, before adding the detail of the jaw and teeth.

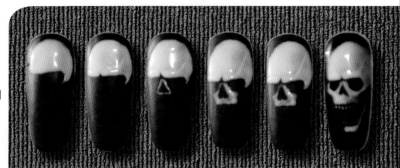

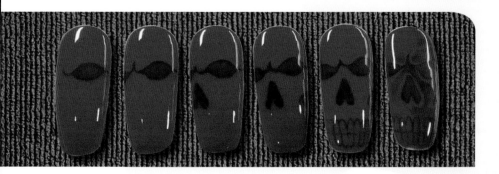

To recreate this spooky design, paint nails in a red shade and when dry use a thin nail art brush and dark blue shade to paint an outline of eye sockets and nose, followed by teeth. Wipe any excess polish from the brush and allow the polish to dry slightly before brushing around the design to shade.

For this tiger design, sponge a grey polish shade onto three areas of the nail and, using a black nail polish and thin nail art brush, add deatailing of the spots, eyes, nose and whiskers. Drag the brush away from the nose outline to create shading and paint within the eye outline in a green shade.

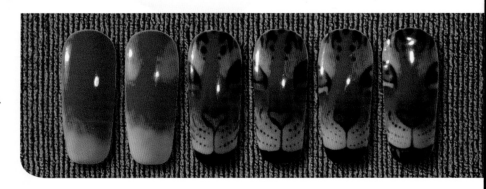

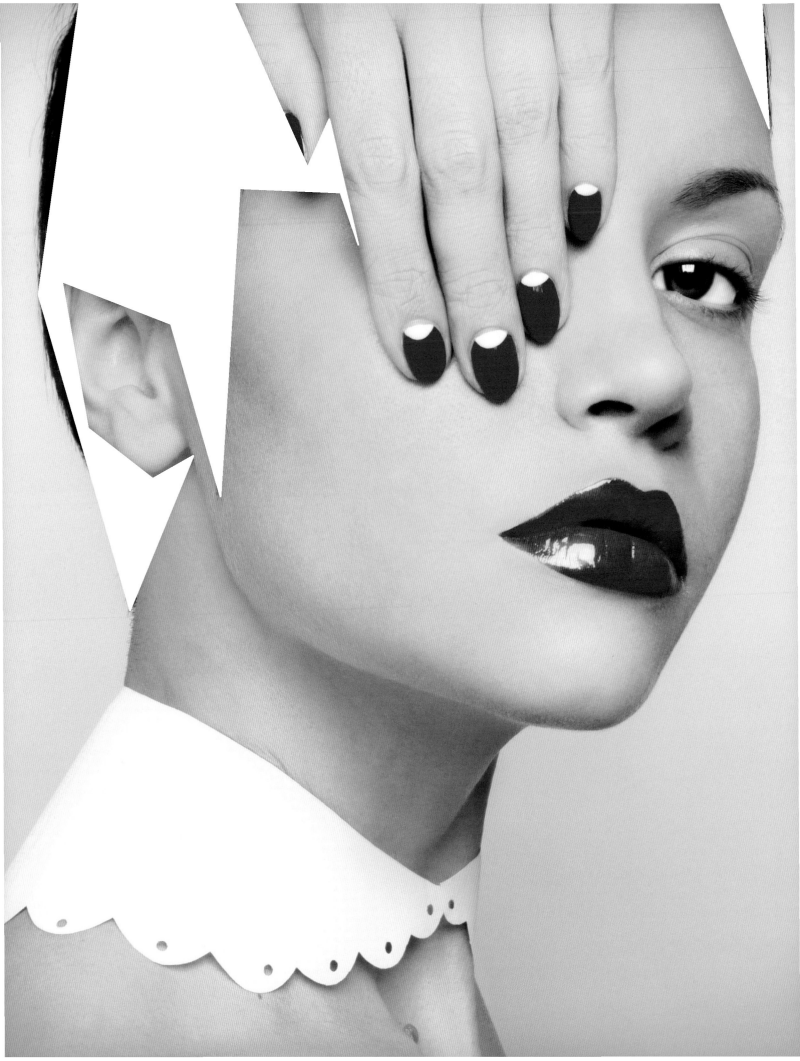

CHAPTER THREE

PERSONAL PREFERENCE

Style in respect of clothing, adornment and attitude can be determined by subculture, practicality or personal taste. It is possibly the boldest and most obvious form of expression in its exposure of the true personality of the individual.

Personal preference can dictate the nail shape and colours worn; some individuals may not like to experiment with design, sporting a classic French or nude shade, while others may choose extended nails in their favourite shades, or in homage to their favourite things.

While many may follow flamboyant fashion trends on a day-to-day basis, nail art can be a subtle way to express personal tastes and passions, which is more practical if the showcasing of dramatic style is not suitable for working life.

Subculture in its various forms can be a huge influence on personal style, from the activities pursued by an individual to the music they listen to, the films they watch and the type of clothes they wear, so it seems fitting that this extends to fingertip design too.

Left *Striking scarlet nails in an almond shape, featuring a white painted half moon design.*

Gothic

The emergence of the modern Gothic subculture in the post-punk era of the early 1980s can be attributed to musical influences. Sinister lyrics inspired by death, isolation and vampire mythology paved the way for dark, theatrical dress styles and make-up choices centred around the colour black.

Favoured dress fabrics include lace, leather, velvet and in recent years PVC, accompanied by silver accessories such as skulls, crosses, bats and magical symbols. Blood-red and deep violet shades are prevalent in Gothic styling, and Gothic styles of architecture and art such as pointed arches, crosses and carvings can also translate into nail design.

Right *Sultry black nails with a freehand painted white cross – iconic of the subculture.*

Below *A dramatic nail image created by Megumi Mizuno, featuring gold, glittery nails with the design extended down the fingertips.*

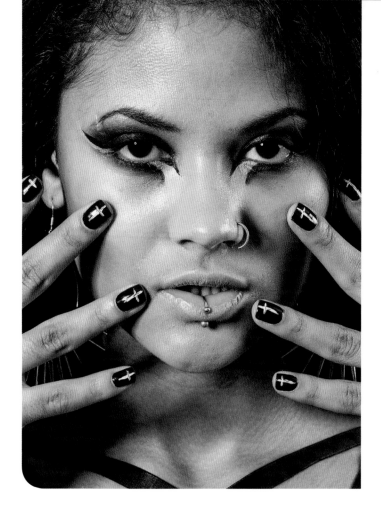

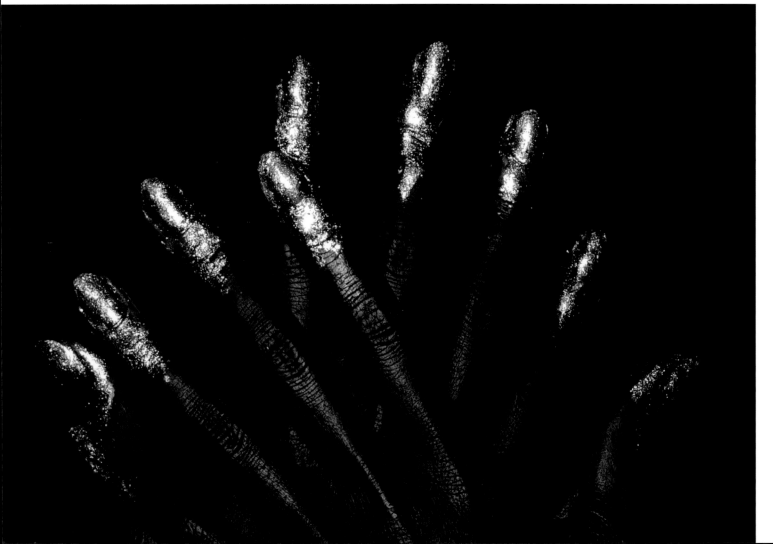

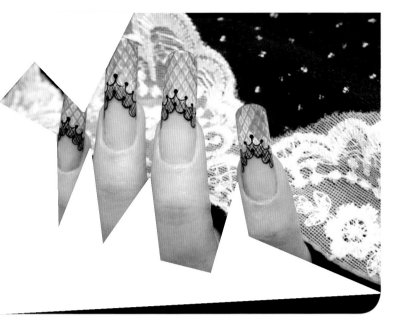

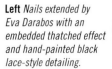

Left *Nails extended by Eva Darabos with an embedded thatched effect and hand-painted black lace-style detailing.*

Right *A dark nail design by Fleury Rose with hand-painted features including blood-effect, spells and spider webs.*

Below left *Nail tips painted in black, red and gold nail shades with stud embellishments and a hand-painted skull design by Megumi Mizuno.*

Below right *Textured nails featuring velvet and a mock-croc effect, finished with diamanté detailing by Sam Biddle.*

Bottom left *Striking scarlet nails with varying red hues and freehand designs in gold and dark red by Sam Biddle.*

Below *Nails painted in black and adorned in a design inspired by Gothic architecture, by Sophie Harris-Greenslade.*

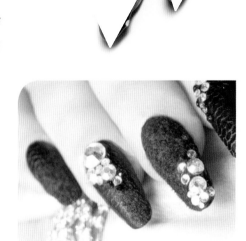

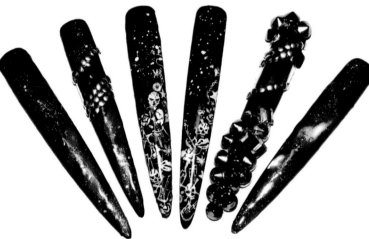

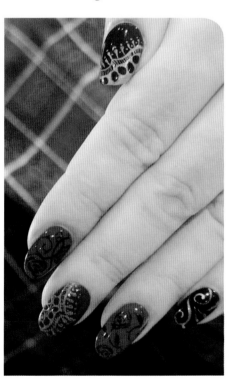

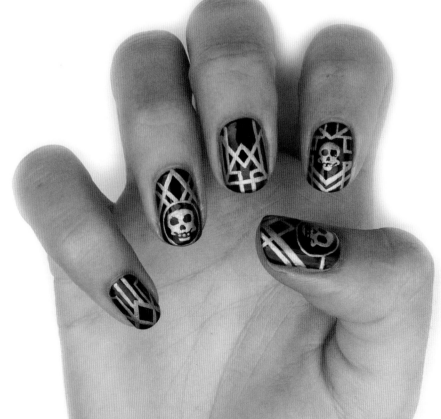

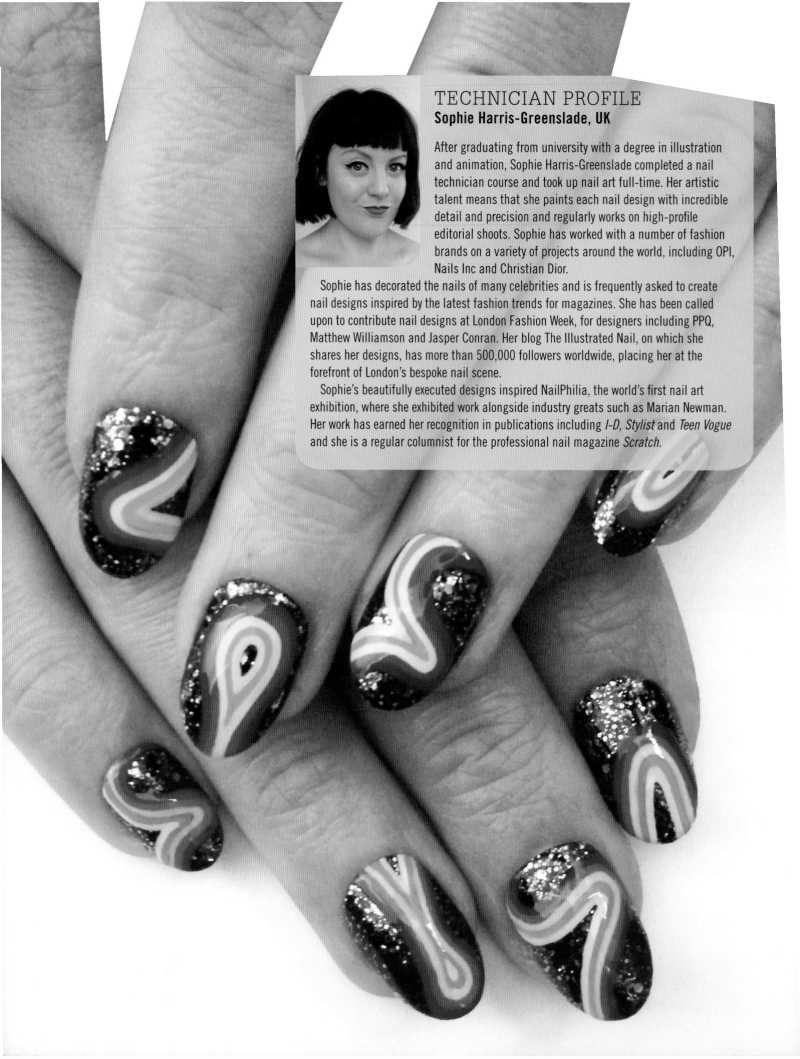

TECHNICIAN PROFILE
Sophie Harris-Greenslade, UK

After graduating from university with a degree in illustration and animation, Sophie Harris-Greenslade completed a nail technician course and took up nail art full-time. Her artistic talent means that she paints each nail design with incredible detail and precision and regularly works on high-profile editorial shoots. Sophie has worked with a number of fashion brands on a variety of projects around the world, including OPI, Nails Inc and Christian Dior.

Sophie has decorated the nails of many celebrities and is frequently asked to create nail designs inspired by the latest fashion trends for magazines. She has been called upon to contribute nail designs at London Fashion Week, for designers including PPQ, Matthew Williamson and Jasper Conran. Her blog The Illustrated Nail, on which she shares her designs, has more than 500,000 followers worldwide, placing her at the forefront of London's bespoke nail scene.

Sophie's beautifully executed designs inspired NailPhilia, the world's first nail art exhibition, where she exhibited work alongside industry greats such as Marian Newman. Her work has earned her recognition in publications including *I-D*, *Stylist* and *Teen Vogue* and she is a regular columnist for the professional nail magazine *Scratch*.

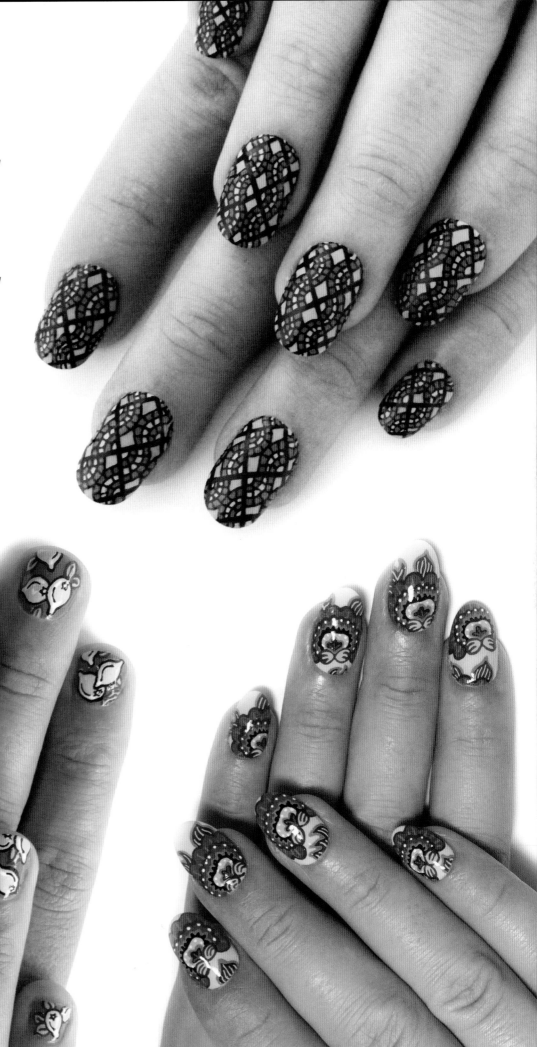

Left *A galaxy-themed nail-art design with random rainbow freehand art.*

Right *An intricate and striking hand-painted nail-art design, reminiscent of a stained-glass window.*

Below *A fruity freehand design in bright nail-polish shades.*

Below right *Oval nails with a bright floral nail-art design randomly positioned across them.*

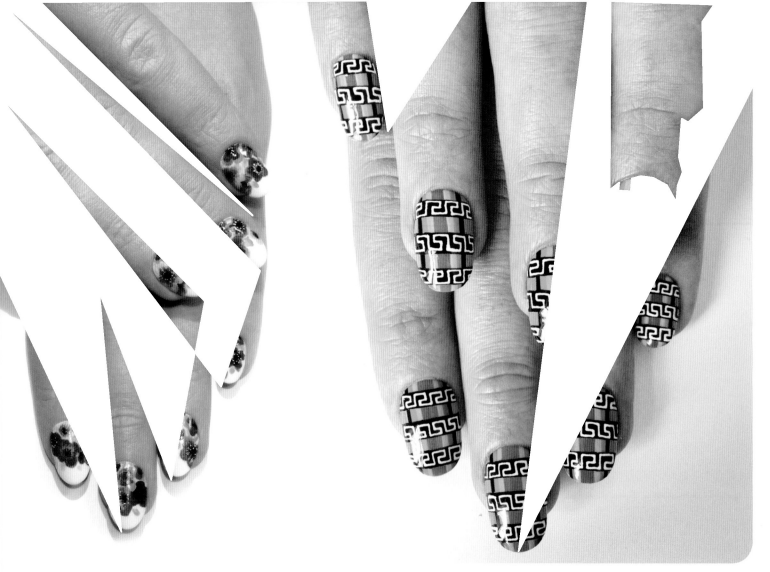

Above *A striking floral nail design on an opaque white polish background.*

Above right *A colourful, stripy nail design with a hand-painted black and white Greek-style overlay.*

Right *Pastel rainbow nails with a freehand white heart-shaped outline, creating a 'negative space' effect.*

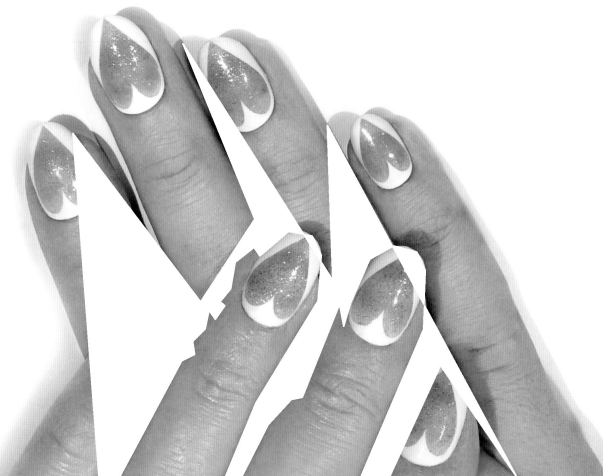

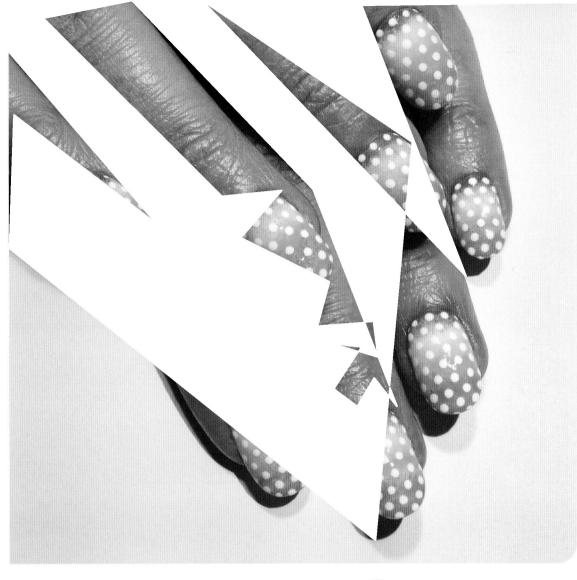

Left *Rainbow nails created by sponging a variety of colours onto the nail, finished with white dots.*

Below *A modern take on the half-moon manicure, with a triangular 'moon' in two bold, striking shades.*

Right *Art-inspired nails with a colourful brushstroke effect.*

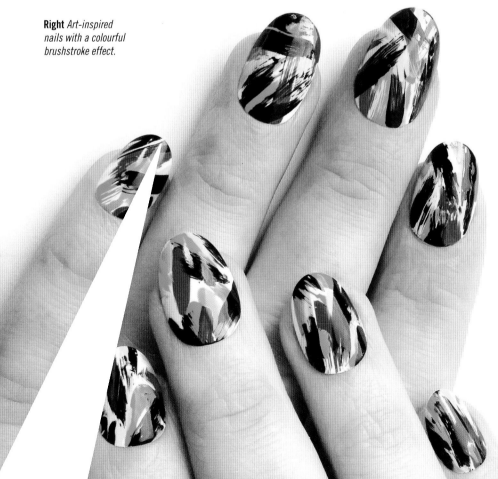

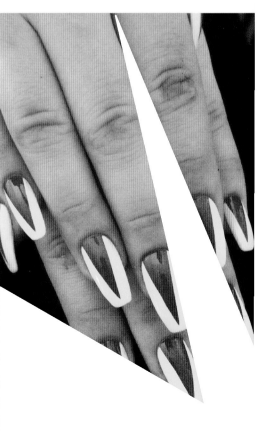

PROJECT: METALLIC CROSS NAILS by Sophie Harris-Greenslade

Sophie Harris-Greenslade demonstrates how to translate the dark shades and cross shapes associated with Gothic style onto nails.

You will need

1 Base coat

2 Black nail polish

3 Top coat

4 Cocktail stick

5 Coloured gems or crystals

6 Scissors

7 Gold metallic striping tape

8 Small silver bullion beads

9 Gold metallic flat stones

10 Bronze striping tape

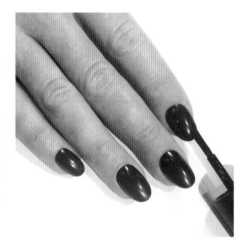

1 Apply base coat and two thin coats of black nail polish to the nails.

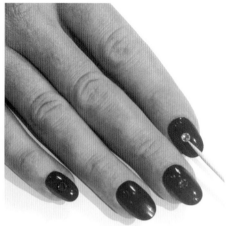

2 Place a small dot of top coat in the centre of all the nails apart from those on the ring fingers. Use a cocktail stick to place a coloured gem on each dot of top coat and press down to secure.

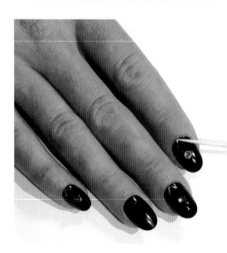

3 Cut two small strips of gold metallic striping tape. Use the top coat and a cocktail stick to place the tape in an upside-down V-shape in the centre of the base of the nail. Repeat on every nail that features a gem.

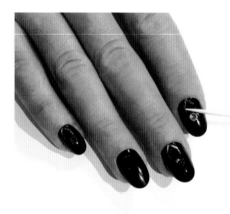

4 Cut two more small strips of striping tape and place vertically on the ends of the V-shape to form the top of the cross.

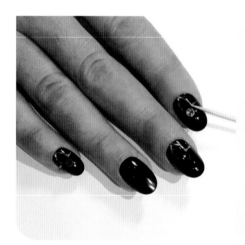

5 Cut two more small strips of gold tape and place horizontally away from the vertical strips.

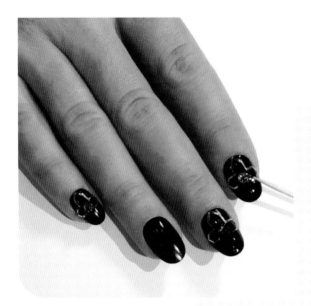

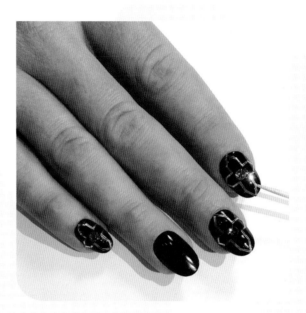

6 Add horizontal V-shapes of gold tape on each side of each gem and two more horizontal strips to form the arms of the cross.

7 Add vertical lines of tape and a V-shape towards the tip of the nail to finish off the cross.

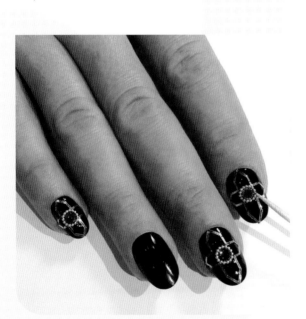

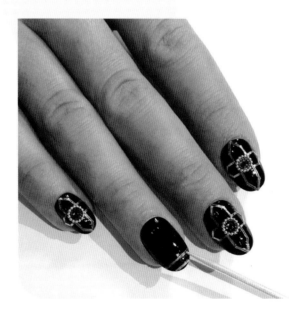

8 Apply a layer of top coat to the eight nails with the cross design and before it dries, add small silver bullion beads around each gem.

9 Apply top coat to the ring finger nails. Cut two strips of gold striping tape and place horizontally at the tip of the nail, leaving a small gap in between.

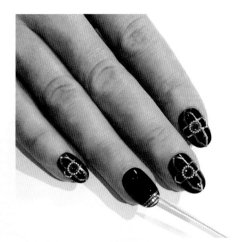

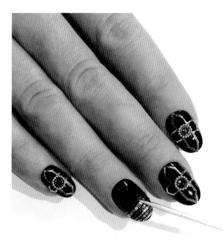

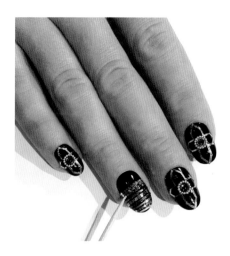

10 In the gap between the tape, add flat gold metallic stones in a line across the nail.

11 Cut two strips of bronze striping tape and place across the nail above the gold tape, leaving a gap in between. Cut small squares from the gold tape and place in a line like a mosaic within the gap.

12 Add another layer of top coat and place gold metallic flat stones in three lines above the bronze tape.

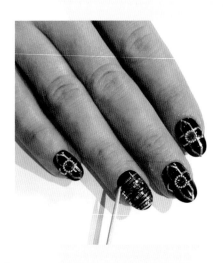

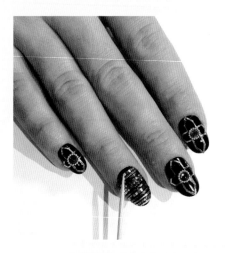

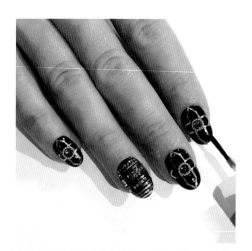

13 Above the lines, add a bronze strip across the nail, followed by a gold one.

14 Cut the gold striping tape to short equal-sized lengths, creating small gold squares. Place in a line across the nail above the bronze and gold strips.

15 Apply a final layer of top coat to all the nails.

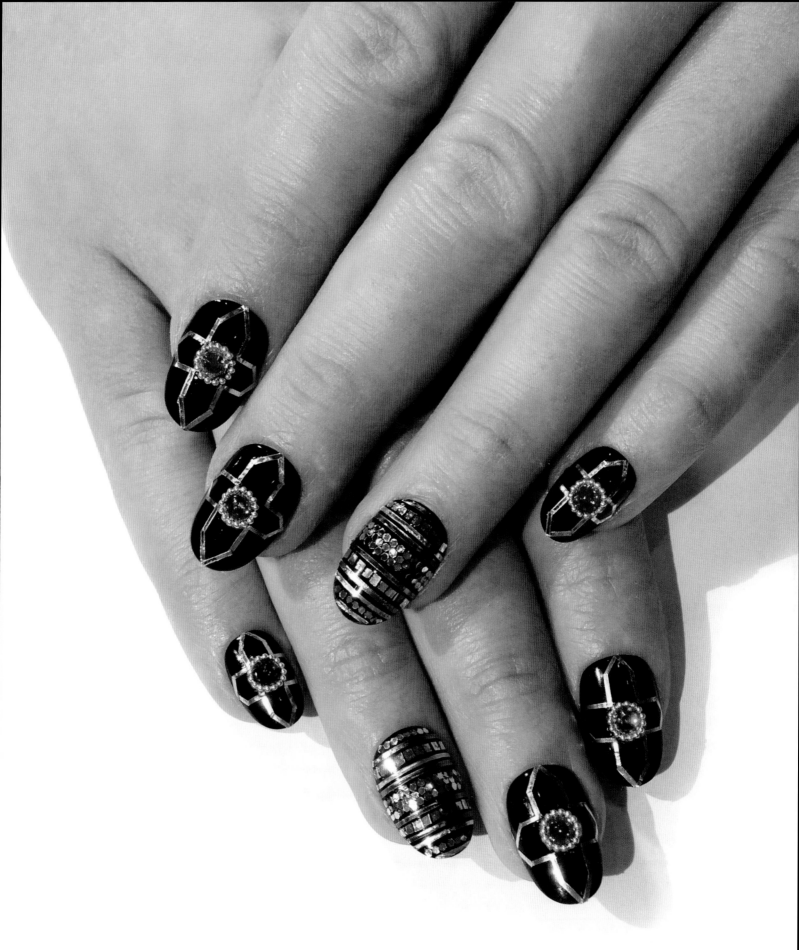

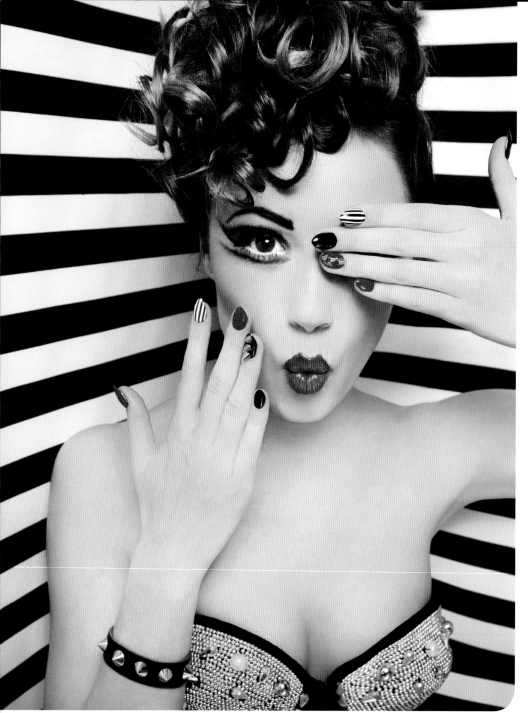

Girly

Gender is a topic of subculture where female sexuality can be expressed through colour and design. Typically girly characteristics include soft pastels – especially pink – and touches of sparkle.

Girly stereotypes have been enhanced through films and toys, with the message that to be girly is to wear floral or pink dresses or skirts and be carefree, with a cute air and positive outlook on life. Activities stereotypically involve shopping and taking time and care over appearance, the latter including nail care, so detailed nail designs to complement clothing are characteristic of this style.

Left *A fun, bright, random nail design featuring pops of fushia pink, monochrome stripes and gold embellishments.*

Below left *Extended almond-shaped nails with a delicate pink shimmer gradient and featuring gold butterfly embellishment by Megumi Mizuno.*

Below *A pretty pink floral detail on a feature nail, created by Eva Darabos.*

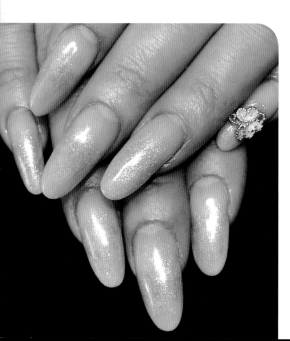

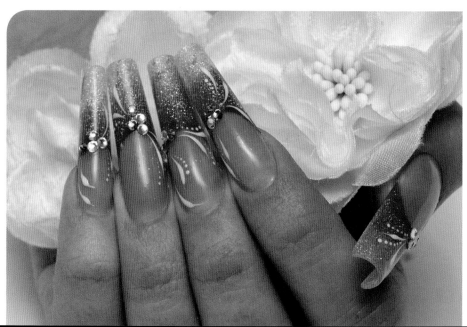

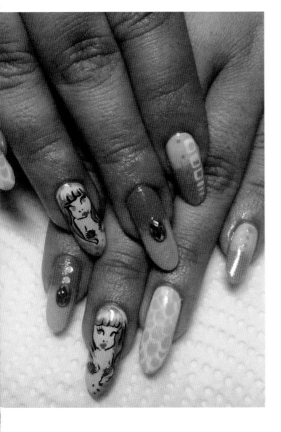

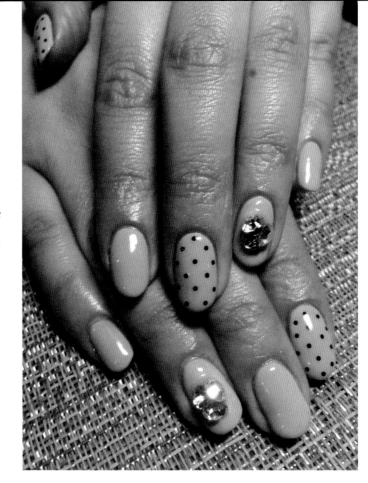

Left *A mermaid-themed nail design in pretty pastel shades, created by Fleury Rose on extended nails.*

Right *Natural nails painted in a delicate lilac shade, featuring polka dots and embellishments on the feature nails by Fleury Rose.*

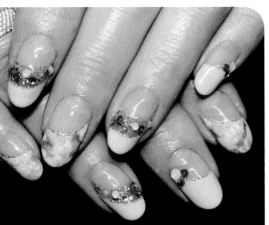

Above *Glossy, oval-shaped nails with pale pink tips and a glittery silver smile line by Megumi Mizuno, featuring eye-catching coloured beads.*

Right *A pink and white marbleized effect by Sam Biddle.*

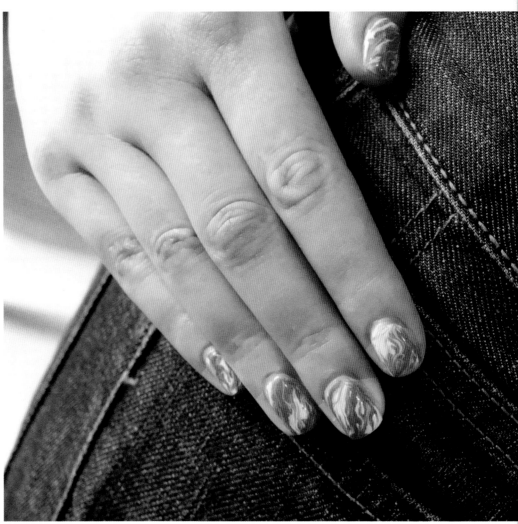

PROJECT: DAISY CHAIN NAILS by Fleury Rose

Fleury Rose shows how to brighten up nails with a fresh, floral and feminine design.

You will need

1 Nail polishes in blue, yellow and black

2 Thin art brush

3 Dotting tool or small brush

4 Top coat

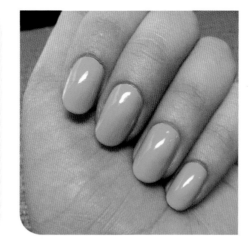

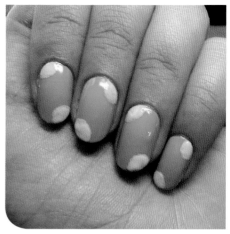

1 Apply two coats of sky-blue polish and allow to dry for 5–10 minutes.

2 Use a pointed brush to dot yellow partial circles on opposite corners of each nail. Clean the brush.

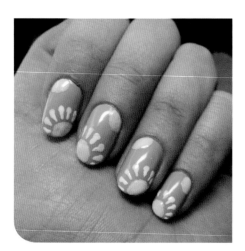

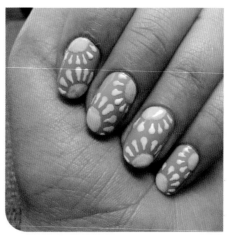

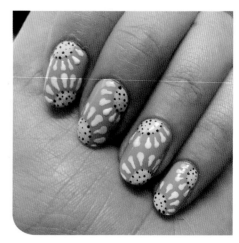

3 Use the brush and white nail polish to create the daisy petals. Dot the colour near the bottom yellow shape and drag outwards. Repeat around the bottom yellow shape on each nail.

4 Repeat Step 3 on the top yellow shape on all the nails.

5 Use a very small brush or dotting tool to add tiny black dots to the centre of the daisy design.

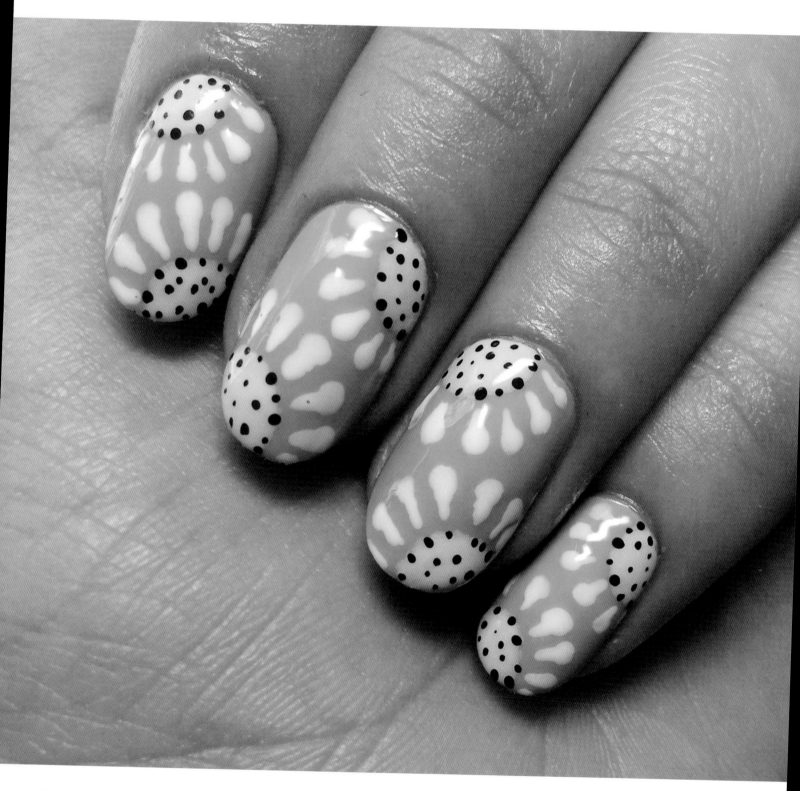

6 Allow the design to dry for 10
minutes and seal with a top coat.

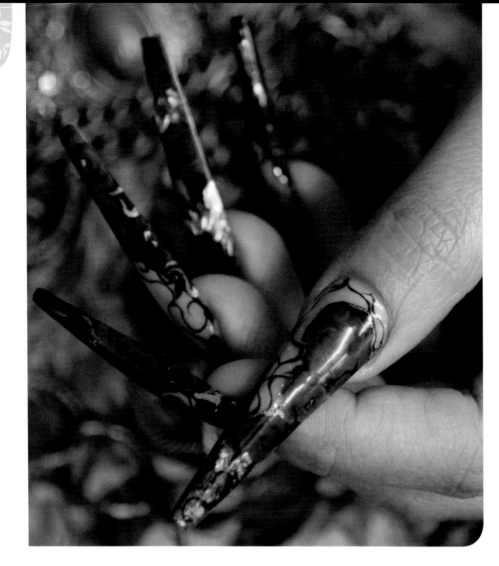

Left *Decadent nail extensions with a hand-painted red rose design, enhanced with black detailing.*

Right *Stiletto-shaped nail extensions with encapsulated pink glittery shades and sculpted 3D flowers, finished with sparkly gems and embellishments.*

Below *Pale pink enhanced nails with pretty floral detailing and gold and silver embellishments.*

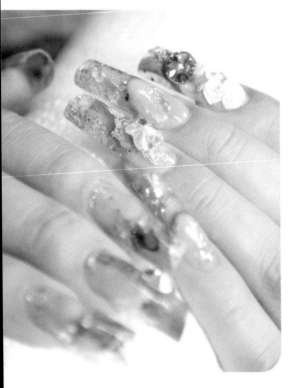

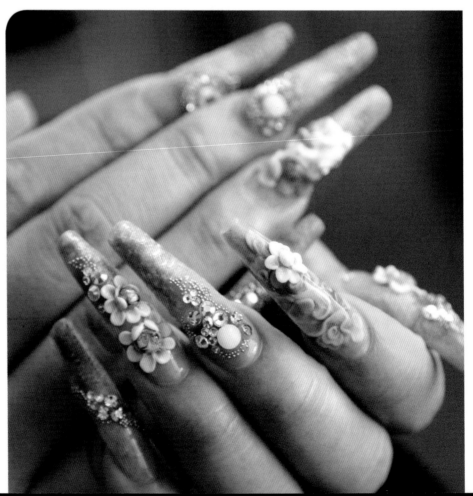

Above *Sparkling and feminine nails featuring gold glitter, mini pearls and 3D embellishments with touches of pink.*

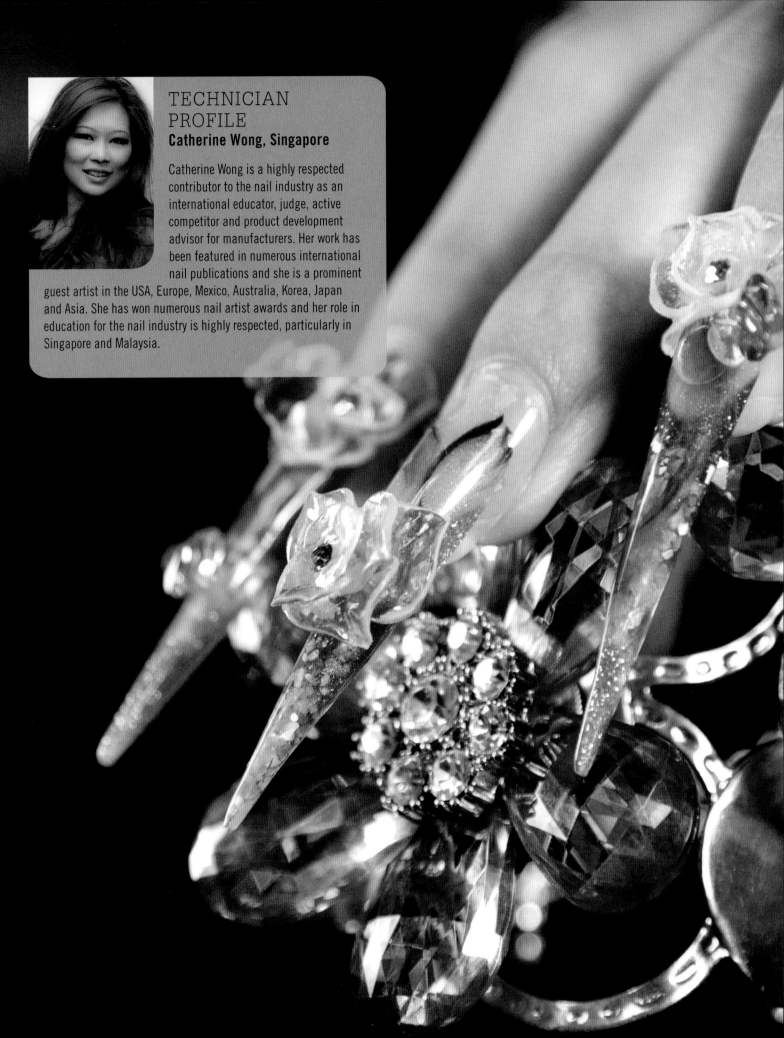

TECHNICIAN PROFILE
Catherine Wong, Singapore

Catherine Wong is a highly respected contributor to the nail industry as an international educator, judge, active competitor and product development advisor for manufacturers. Her work has been featured in numerous international nail publications and she is a prominent guest artist in the USA, Europe, Mexico, Australia, Korea, Japan and Asia. She has won numerous nail artist awards and her role in education for the nail industry is highly respected, particularly in Singapore and Malaysia.

Glamorous

A glamorous style conjures up imagery of lavish gowns, designer apparel, a well-groomed appearance and plenty of sparkle. Celebrity culture is responsible for inspiration, especially the Hollywood glamour style, where actresses and actors are given a particular look to separate them from the masses and turn them into idolized figures.

Elegance is a key characteristic of glamour, and can be enhanced through nail design with an almond or extended stiletto shape. Scarlet and other shades of red are commonly associated with the style, along with the classic black, gold and silver so typical of glamorous nail designs. Glamour should be effortless in appearance and present a particularly luxurious impression, so consider straightforward designs in shades that befit the style.

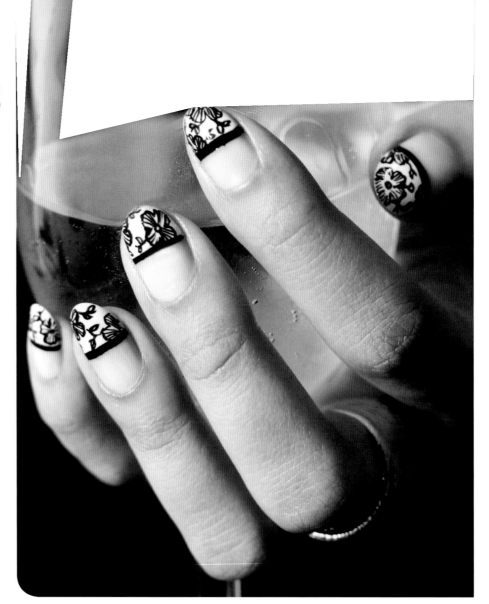

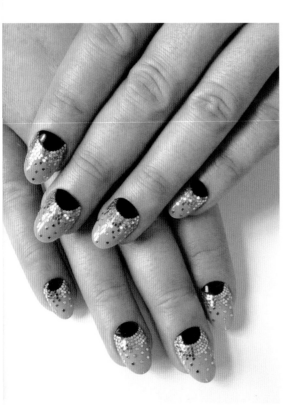

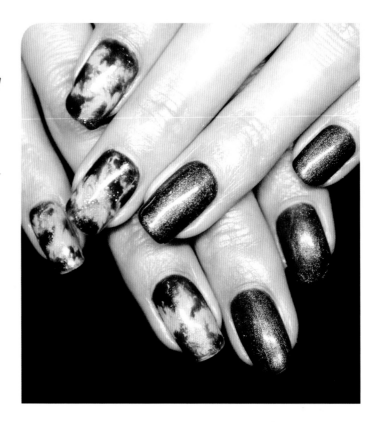

Above *An elegant nail look slightly influenced by the French manicure. Featuring a timeless monochrome floral design painted freehand by Ami Vega.*

Left *An elegant half moon nail design with gold embellishments. Created by Sophie Harris-Greenslade on nails shaped to the feminine almond.*

Right *Elegant, squoval-shaped nails by Megumi Mizuno, featuring a combination of tortoiseshell effect and bronze, shimmery nails.*

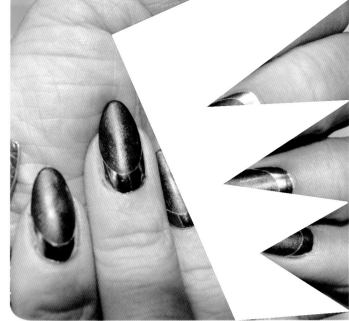

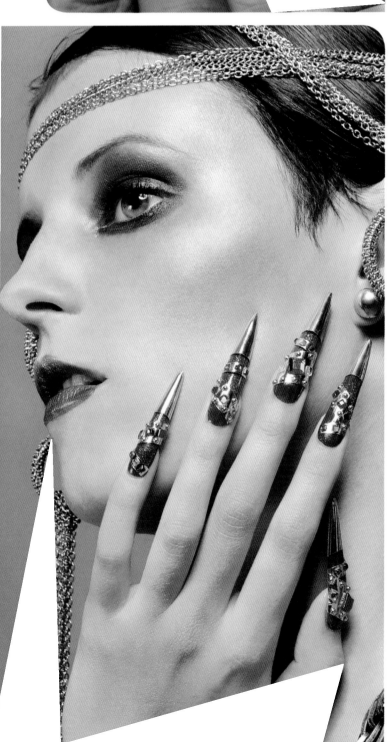

Left *Matte, marble-effect nails shaped to a feminine almond, with glamorous gold foil detailing by the cuticle area by Megumi Mizuno.*

Top right *Gold, shimmery nails by Fleury Rose, with a black hand-painted effect and crystal-encrusted ring fingers.*

Right *Hand-painted lace-effect nails among nude nails with a black halo design, by Fleury Rose.*

Bottom left *An unusual extended nail design with embellishments and gold foil tips by Megumi Mizuno.*

Below *Pretty gold glitter nail tips and an assortment of jewelled embellishments, designed and crafted by Megumi Mizuno.*

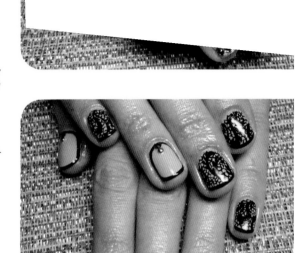

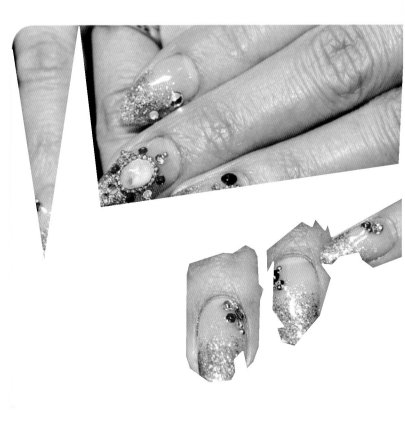

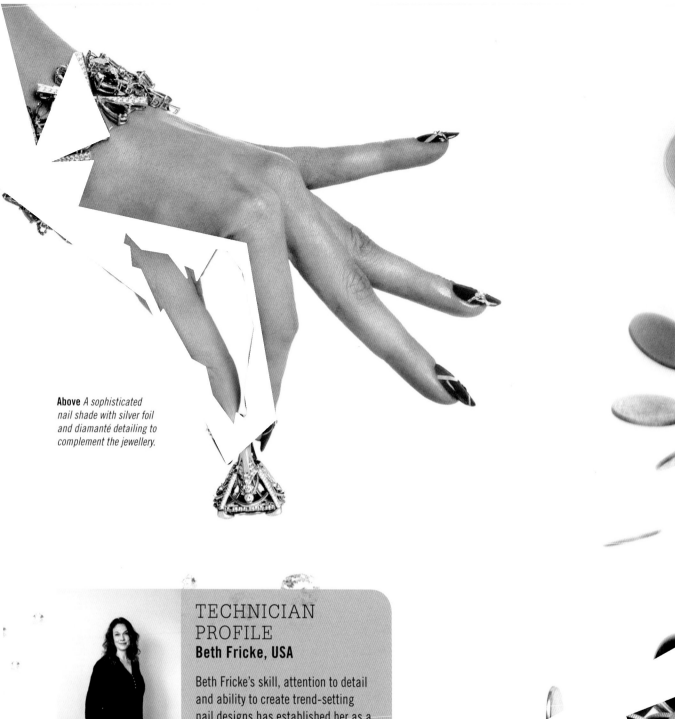

Above *A sophisticated nail shade with silver foil and diamanté detailing to complement the jewellery.*

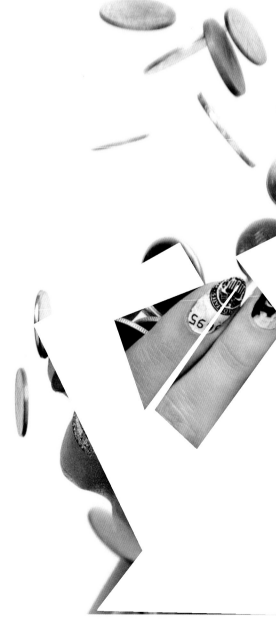

TECHNICIAN PROFILE
Beth Fricke, USA

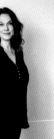

Beth Fricke's skill, attention to detail and ability to create trend-setting nail designs has established her as a prominent manicurist in the fashion, beauty and entertainment industries. After qualifying as a nail technician at the age of 18 in her hometown of Kansas City, Beth worked in a number of salons while studying journalism and radio and television production at university.

Combining her background in manicuring and production, Beth relocated to Los Angeles, where she spent five years in music video and commercials production. Since then she has expanded her portfolio and her nail work has appeared on the front covers of magazines including *Elle*, *Harper's Bazaar*, *Glamour* and *Nylon*. Beth has contributed advice on emerging nail trends and nail care to a number of publications and has developed an impressive celebrity roster that includes Drew Barrymore, Heidi Klum, Miranda Kerr and Mariah Carey.

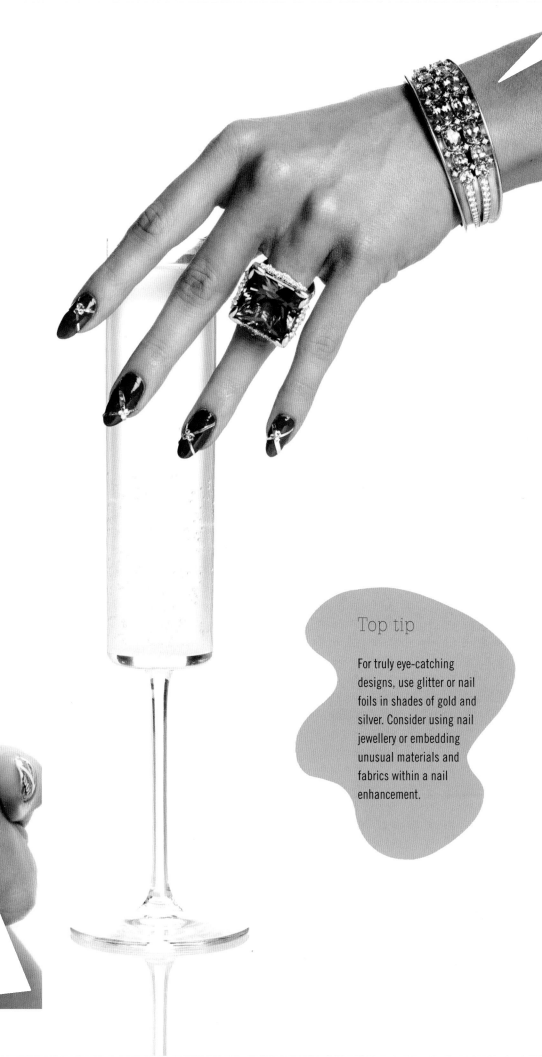

Right *Elegant oval-shaped nails in a block shade with silver detailing.*

Below *US dollar nail wraps applied to oval-shaped nails.*

Top tip

For truly eye-catching designs, use glitter or nail foils in shades of gold and silver. Consider using nail jewellery or embedding unusual materials and fabrics within a nail enhancement.

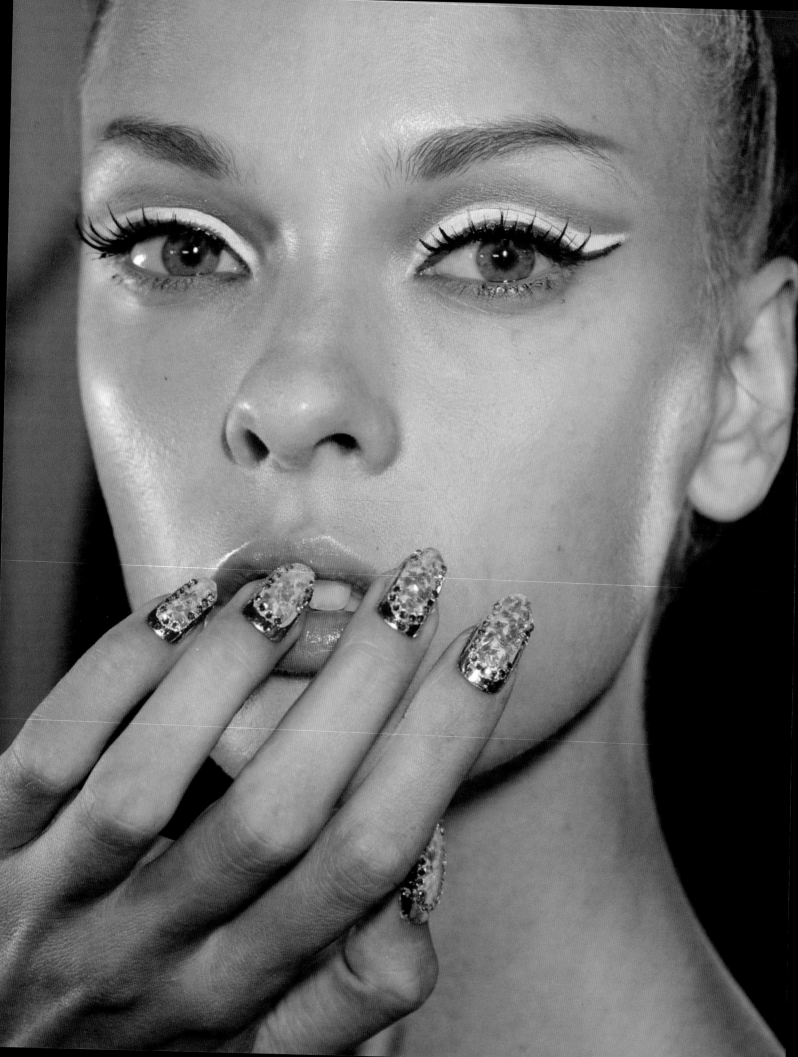

CHAPTER FOUR
FASHION

When a designer begins to develop a new collection, he or she tends to have a muse in mind – a woman or man of certain character, who has travelled a particular path in life and enjoys specific activities. The designer then finds fabrics and textures to suit the traits of the muse, constructing designs to convey his or her characteristics.

When showcasing the finished clothing collection, the model, hair, make-up and shoes are all taken into consideration, as well as nail colour and design. While nude or plain nails have been preferred historically in order not to detract attention from the clothing, in recent years designers have embraced nail colour and art as a way to complete the overall look.

Fashion designers meet with hair, make-up, nail and styling teams in the weeks leading up to the presentation of their collection in order to construct ideas for the way in which all elements should come together and showcase the personality of the collection to its full potential. After these collections have been shown to set the precedent for the next fashion season, they are translated into more wearable, affordable fashions and then magazines display the clothing, make-up, hair and nail looks that will be on trend for the season.

How an individual chooses to interpret a fashion trend is a matter of choice. It can be followed in an extreme way, replicating the trend through every medium possible, or in a subtle way, through wearing a different make-up shade or nail look.

Left *Striking yellow and gold nails with embellishments by CND to complement The Blonds Spring/Summer collection and the make-up style.*

Classic and Chic

While the fashion world has become noticeably more experimental with nail design, many designers still prefer nude, bare or French nails for models when showcasing their collections. Nude nails or a French manicure give the illusion of an extension of the fingertips, offering a clean, well-groomed finish that complements clothing of any colour. These styles, or a plain, well-filed nail, perhaps with clear polish, are excellent options for everyday wear, particularly in the professional world, because of their subtlety. The shape can be tailored to the type of woman the designer wants to portray, or the practical needs of the wearer; square or almond for a feminine, casual, everyday appearance or pointed and extended for a more fierce, powerful look.

In stark contrast, plain black nails with either a glossy or matte finish offer a chic nail look. While not suited to pale skin tones (unless the Gothic look is the aim), black nails – like an iconic little black dress – are sophisticated and the shade also complements most ensembles. It is most popular in the winter months, while an opaque white nail finish achieves a similar effect in the summer.

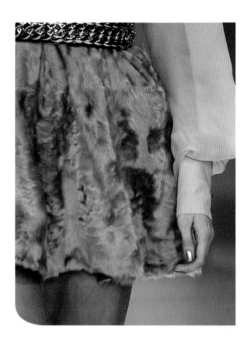

Above *Nails with a rounded edge painted by Antonio Sacripante in a golden polish to complement accessories at the spring/summer Genny show.*

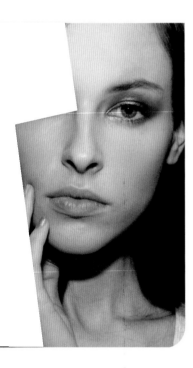

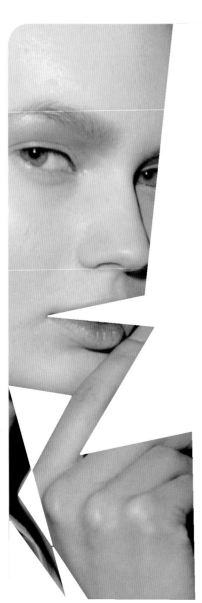

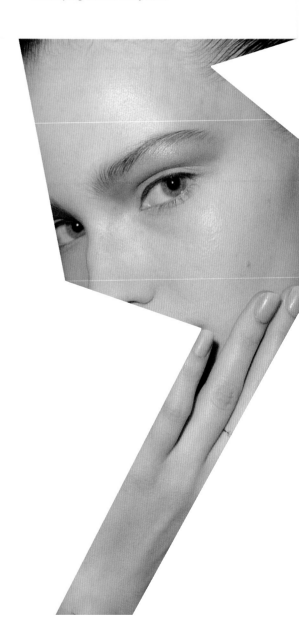

Above *Golden nails for the Genny spring/summer collection by Antonio Sacripante.*

Right
Models showcase a natural nail design to complement the skin tone by CND for Alexander Wang's Autumn/ Winter collection.

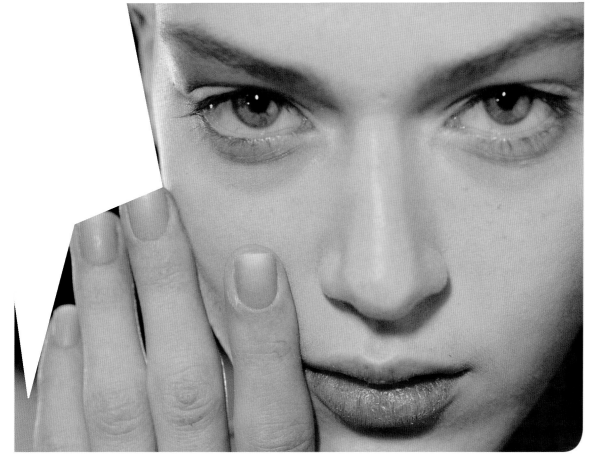

Left *A model displays the subtle nail shades selected by CND for Alexander Wang's Autumn/Winter collection.*

Below *Nails in a soft square shape in a mottled shade of nude created by CND for Alexander Wang's Autumn/Winter collection.*

Below left *Natural nails with a slight gloss, give the illusion of elongated fingers. These nails, designed by Antonio Sacripante and team for Gianfranco Ferre, Spring/ Summer, ensure the focus remains on the clothing in the collection.*

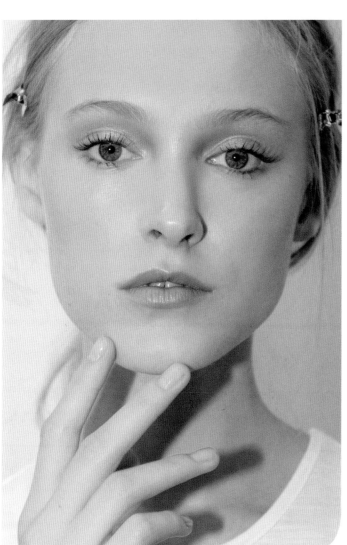

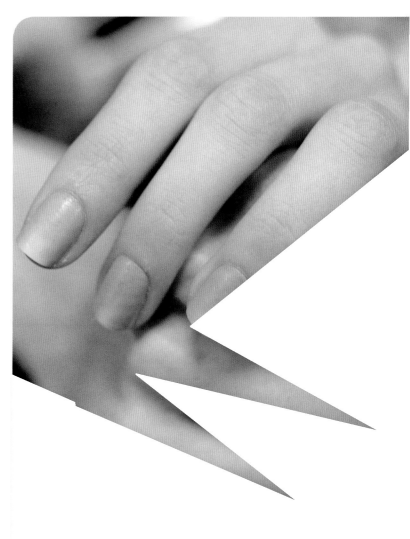

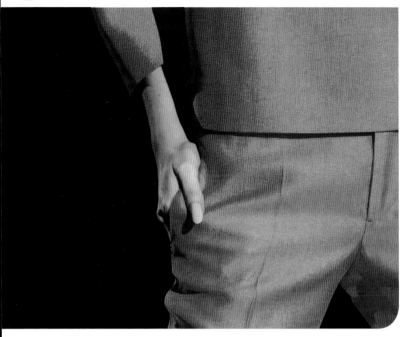

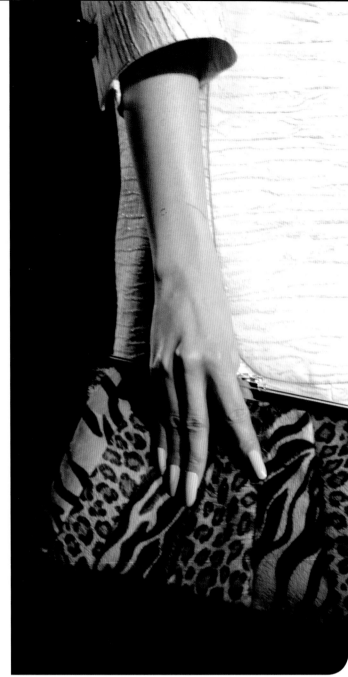

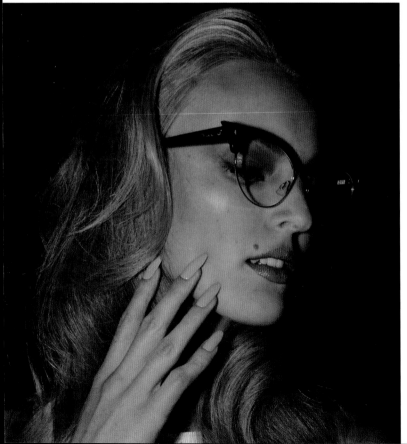

Image Gallery

Above left *Pretty pink almond-shaped nails by Antonio Sacripante and team were designed to contrast with the collection at DSquared2 Spring/Summer.*

Above *Close-up of the feminine nail design from the DSquared2 Spring/Summer collection, conceptualized by Antonio Sacripante.*

Left *Another close-up of nails from the DSquared2 show. The pale pink of the nails added a subtle, feminine touch to the collection, which featured occasional bright hues.*

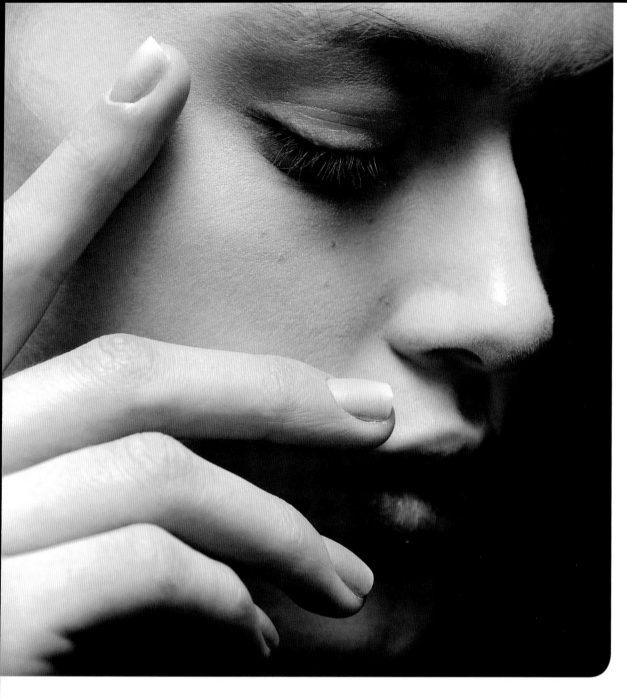

Left and Below Left
*Short, natural-looking
nails created by a team
of CND nail technicians
for Alexander Wang to
complement the subtle
make-up hues of his
Autumn/Winter collection.*

Below centre *Feminine,
pale pink nails contrasted
with the exuberant prints
and bold shades by Antonio
Sacripante and team for
DSquared2 Spring/Summer.*

Below *A pretty gold
shimmer polish was used
by Antonio Sacripante
and team to complement
elements of the fabrics
used in the Genny Spring/
Summer fashion showcase.*

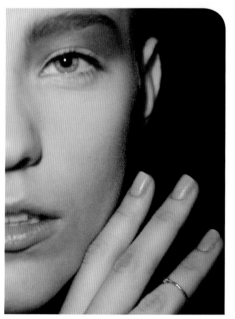

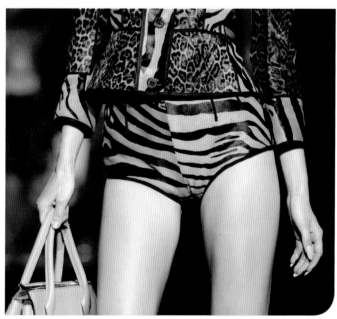

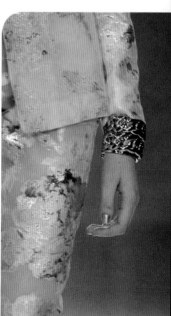

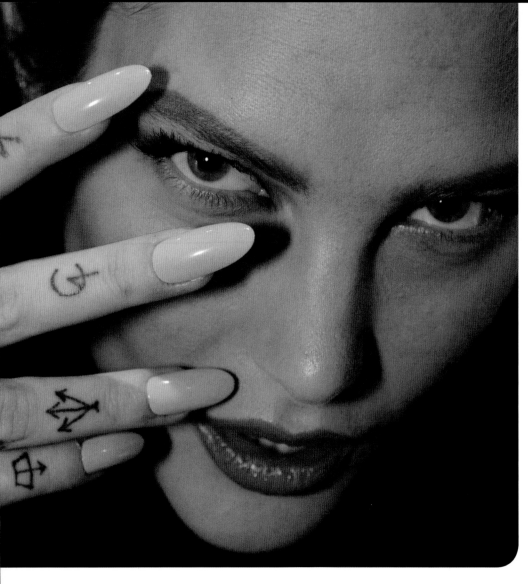

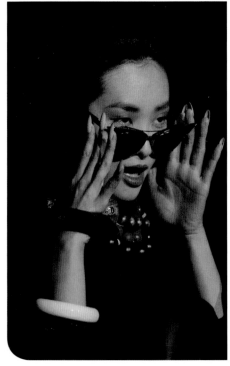

Left *An elongated nail design conceptualized by Antonio Sacripante for DSquared2 Spring/ Summer collection.*

Above *A model showcases the elegant, almond nails at DSquared2.*

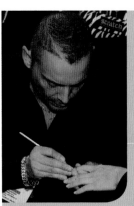

TECHNICIAN PROFILE
Antonio Sacripante, Italy

Antonio Sacripante stepped into the nail industry after graduating from university, translating his studies of polymers into a keen interest in nail products and nail art. After he won a number of nail competitions, his creative streak led him into the fashion field and he has headed up nail teams for shows at Milan Fashion Week since 2007, including Les Copains and DSquared2. He holds the title of Dean of Education for one of the world's biggest nail brands, Hand and Nail Harmony, and runs his own training academy in Italy, as well as working with celebrities and as a nail competition judge and trainer.

Antonio appears regularly on Russia's World Fashion Channel as a nail fashion expert and in 2013 he had a nail design on 12 nail tips showcased in an exhibition of Italian culture in the USA, entitled The Cutting Age. Drawing on his expertise in miniature nail design, Antonio crafted a woodland scene overlooking the sea, using nail products alongside natural materials such as oak bark and dried flowers.

'Each time I am asked to create nails for a designer's collection, I make sure that I spend a lot of time talking with them to find the perfect nail art to match the mood and the philosophy of their collection. It's always a joint effort; designers know what they want on their catwalks and as a nail artist I must find a way to give them what they need, with some surprising twists.' Antonio Sacripante

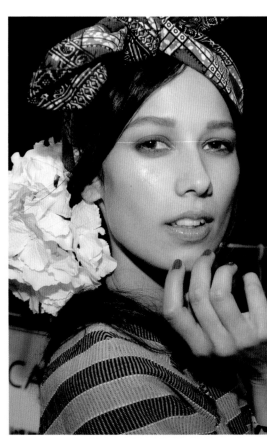

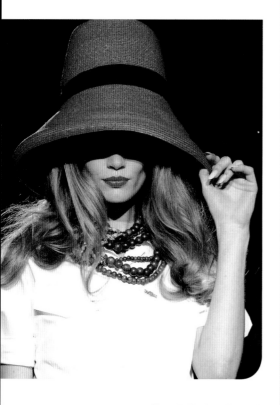

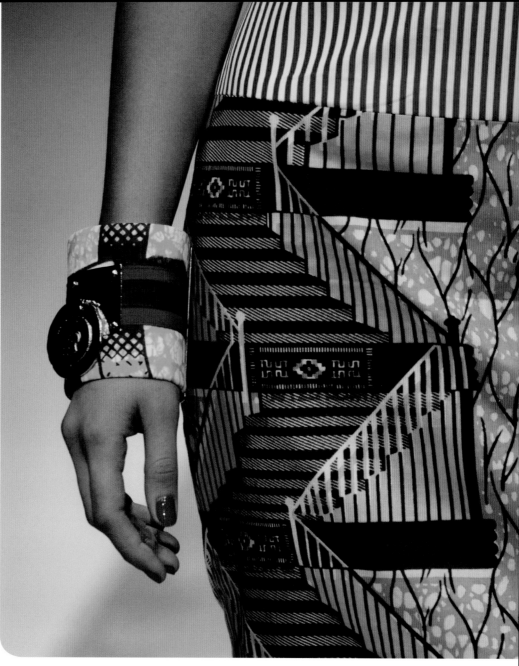

Above *Pale, almond nails at DSquared2 allowed the bold fabrics in the collection to maintain focus.*

Right *Bold, fuchsia nails complemented busy prints at the Stella Jean Spring/ Summer show.*

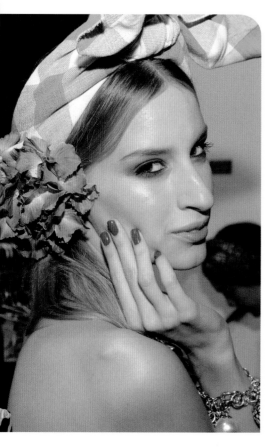

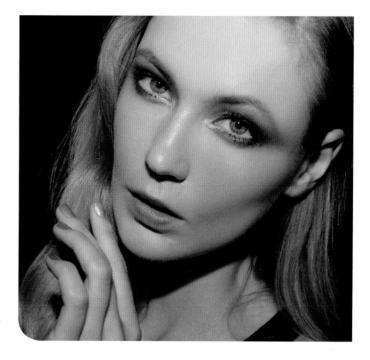

Left *Models at Stella Jean show the bright nail shade used to complete the bold look.*

Right *Shimmery, gold nail polish on natural nails for the Genny Spring/Summer fashion showcase.*

Prints and Patterns

Wearing a fashionable nail shade or translating an element of a collection into nail art is an affordable way to honour a trend. Whether the design or the texture of a fashionable fabric is selected, it can be echoed on nails using nail art tools, polishes and even stencils.

When working with high-fashion designers, nail teams conceptualize several ideas for the designer's choosing which can complement the colours of the clothing or replicate a pattern or element of the design. Nail shape can also play a pivotal role in expressing the personality of the muse.

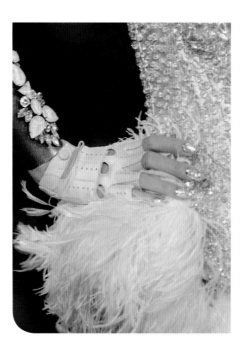

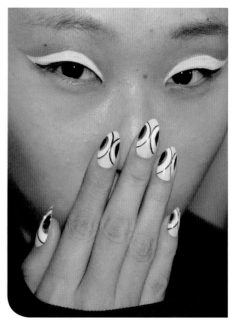

Above *Bright yellow, crystal-embellished nails by CND perfectly matched one of the ensembles designed by The Blonds for the Spring/Summer collection.*

Above *A bright, statement nail design by CND for The Blonds captured elements of the make-up and the Spring/Summer collection.*

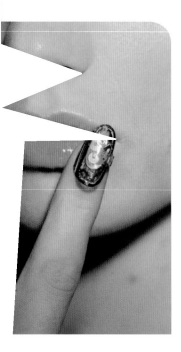

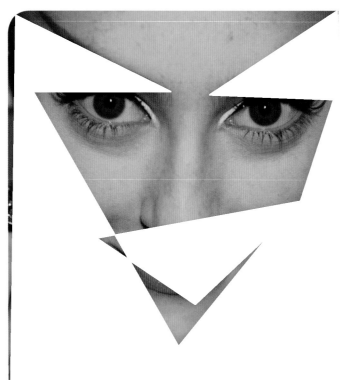

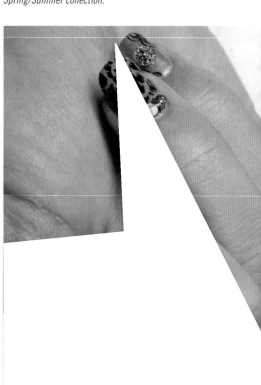

Above *Close up of one of the many nail designs by CND for The Blonds.*

Right *Random, embellished metallic nails by CND for The Blonds Spring/Summer fashion showcase.*

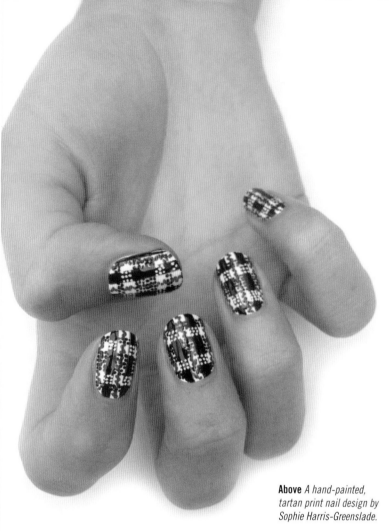

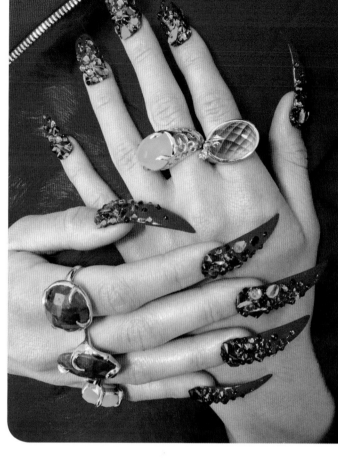

Above *A hand-painted, tartan print nail design by Sophie Harris-Greenslade.*

Left *Nails inspired by varied fabrics and textures with a recurring gold theme, hand-painted by Astrowifey.*

Above *Extravagant scarlet nail extensions shaped to a point and embellished with blue crystals by Sophie Harris-Greenslade to complement a coat.*

Below *Close up of hand-painted floral nails by Sophie Harris-Greenslade, inspired by elements of the model's clothing.*

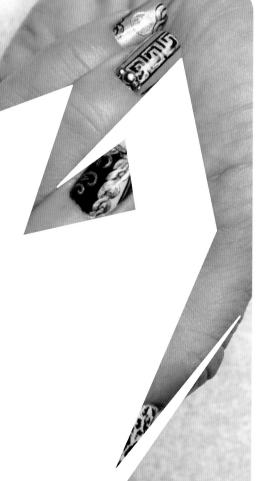

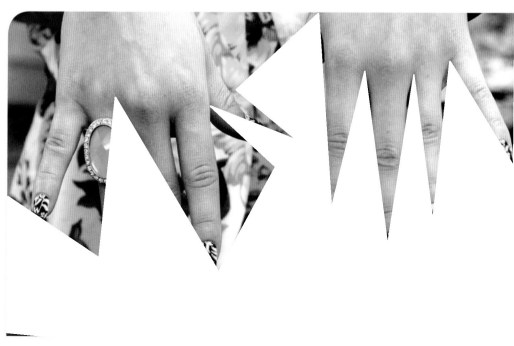

FASHION AND NAILS CASE STUDY: Michael van der Ham and CND

Professional nail-care company CND was chosen by designer Michael van der Ham to create artistic nail designs to complement his Spring/Summer 2014 collection. The inspiration for van der Ham's collection came from *Farm* by Jackie Nickerson, a photographic book focusing on the beautiful clothing worn by Zimbabwean farmworkers. While the fabric shades developed into worn, edgy pastels and bold yellow and navy hues, van der Ham still reinforced his signature style, matching unusual textures with subtle cuts to present his muse: a spontaneous, free-spirited woman with a feminine and eclectic edge.

CND co-founder Jan Arnold was shown the initial designs and fabrics and discussed nail ideas at length with van der Ham before she and an elite team of CND nail artists created four final nail looks for the models. These nail designs were soft in focus, inspired by a romantic and impressionistic garden to present a whimsical, almost ethereal style that reflected van der Ham's muse. To represent the free, eclectic attitude of the woman in mind, the hand-painted nails were shaped in a casual, easy-to-wear way and the colour combinations were yellow and grey, teal and black, deep navy and purple, and pink, grey and coral.

Below *A model walks the runway at Michael van der Ham's Spring/Summer showcase.*

Right *Varied prints and rich, textured fabrics at the collection showcased elements of Michael van der Ham's muse and served to inspire the nail design by CND.*

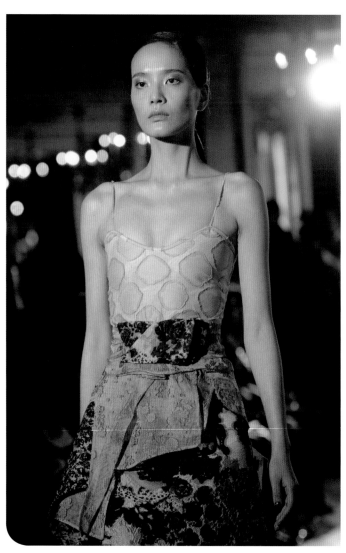

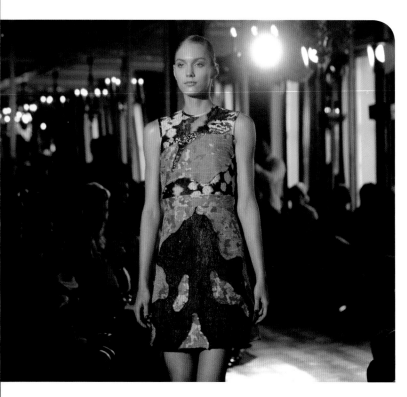

Below *A close-up of the fabric used, with nails by CND to complement it.*

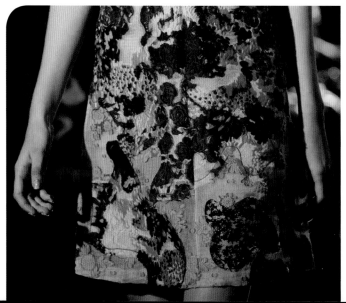

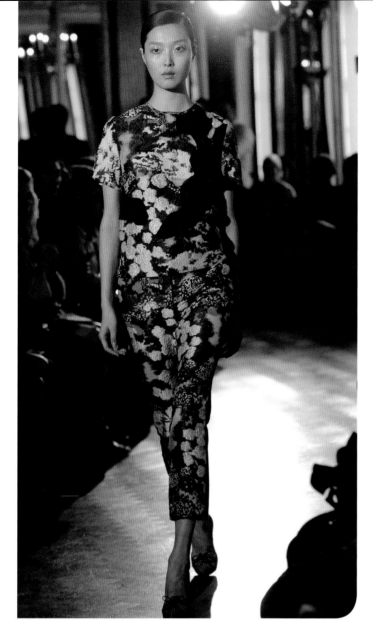

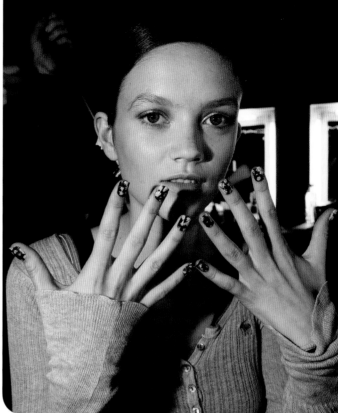

Above A close up of the yellow and black nails created by CND for Michael van der Ham, complementing the textures and fabrics of his Spring/Summer collection.

Above A model walks the runway wearing one of the four nail designs created by CND for Michael van der Ham's Spring/Summer collection.

Below A model is filmed backstage, displaying one of the four nail looks that were designed to complement van der Ham's collection.

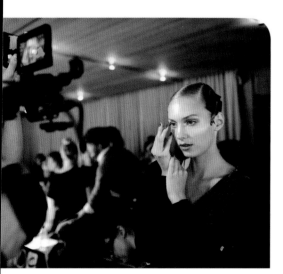

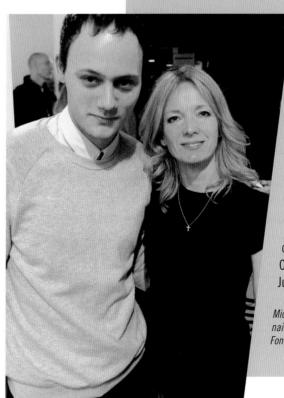

STYLE FILE
Michael van der Ham

Born in the Netherlands, Michael van der Ham is a graduate of the MA fashion course at Central Saint Martins College of Art and Design in London. He has been showing his collections at London Fashion Week since 2009, and is one of the recipients of the British Fashion Council's NEWGEN sponsorship. He is recognized by the British Fashion Awards for his ready-to-wear designs, which bring together elegant silhouettes and a unique blend of fabrics and textures.

Michael was approached by costume designer Suttirat Larlarb and director Danny Boyle to design 250 costumes for one of the sequences of the London Olympics opening ceremony in July 2012.

Michael van der Ham with the lead nail technician for the show, Amanda Fontanarrosa of CND.

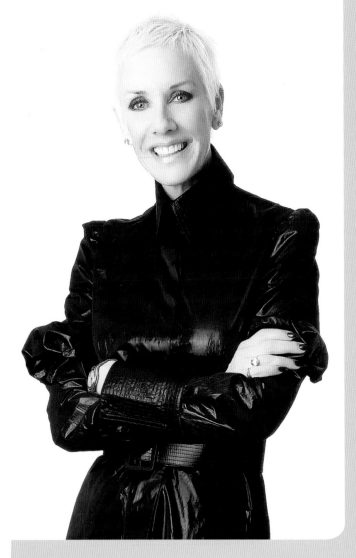

STYLE FILE
Jan Arnold

Jan Arnold is the co-founder of CND (formerly Creative Nail Design) and her experience as a brand engineer has contributed to its success as a worldwide company. Her personal sense of style makes her the high-fashion face behind the brand and she is often referred to as 'Fashion's first lady of nails'.

Jan is a key link between the professional nail industry and international high fashion and has pioneered custom nail styles for top designers all over the world, including Alexander Wang, Michael van der Ham, Jason Wu, Phillip Lim and The Blonds. Jan credits nails as 'the ultimate fashion accessory – the perfect punctuation to an outfit and personality and a defining statement to style'.

'In recent years, mainstream designers have become more open-minded to experimenting with colour, design and texture. Nail art is finally becoming mainstream because it is an easily obtainable runway statement. In the past few years, the widely acknowledged definition "nail art" has morphed from literal stars and rainbows to more sophisticated designs which are now considered nail fashion.'
Jan Arnold

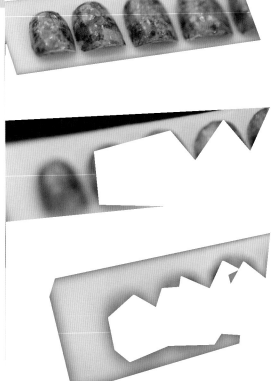

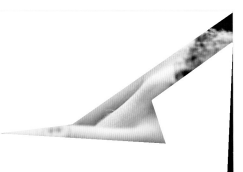

Left *Close-up of the nails being shaped to fit the models' nails at Michael van der Ham, Spring/ Summer.*

Right *One of the four nail designs created on tips by CND for the collection, ready to adhere to models' nails.*

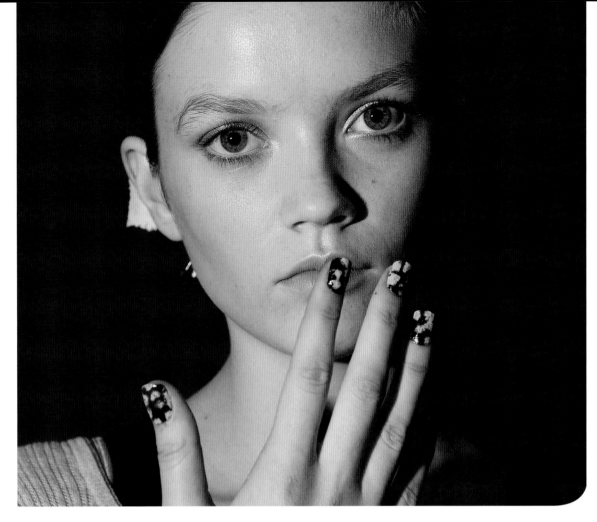

Left *Close-up of one of the four impressionistic nail designs by CND for Michael van der Ham Spring/ Summer, created using sponging and layering techniques with CND Vinylux.*

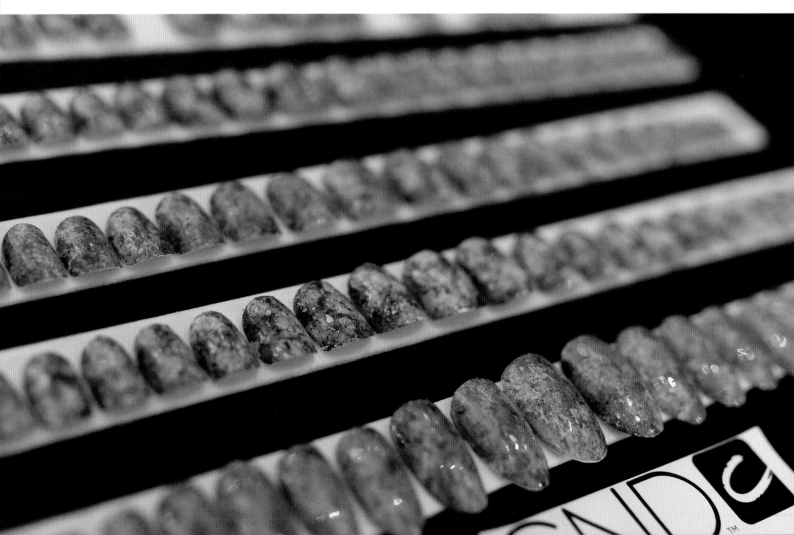

PROJECT: NAILS FOR MICHAEL VAN DER HAM, SPRING/SUMMER COLLECTION

by Amanda Fontanarrosa

Amanda Fontanarrosa, education ambassador and media spokesperson for CND, shows how to imitate the nail looks from Michael van der Ham's Spring/Summer London Fashion Week showcase.

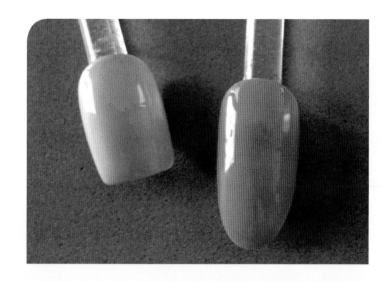

1 Shape the nails into either an almond or square shape using a natural nail file and apply two coats of your chosen shade. Pictured: a square-shaped nail painted with CND Vinylux in Cityscape and an almond-shaped nail using CND Vinylux in Gotcha.

2 With the make-up sponge pieces, drip a small amount of four or five chosen nail shades onto a tray. Pictured: CND Vinylux shades in Asphalt, Lobster Roll, Cityscape, Gotcha and Married to the Mauve.

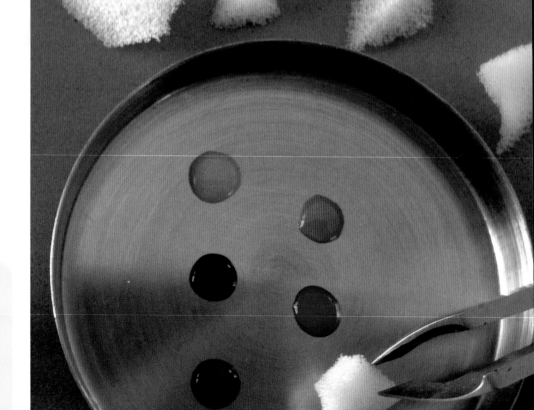

You will need

1 Four or five nail shades

2 Make-up sponge, cut into small pieces

3 Tweezers

4 Top coat

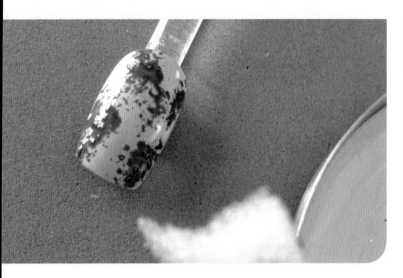

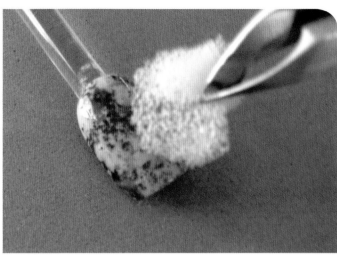

3 Using the sponge and some tweezers, sponge your chosen first shade randomly onto all 10 nails. Allow them to dry.

4 Choose a second colour and again, sponge randomly onto all 10 nails. Continue with the remaining shades, allowing each colour to dry before applying the next to avoid smearing. Apply top coat to finish.

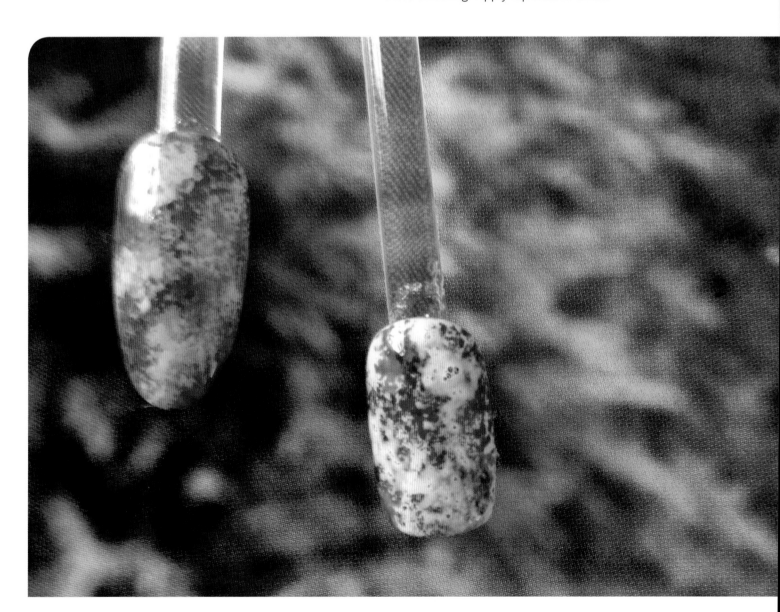

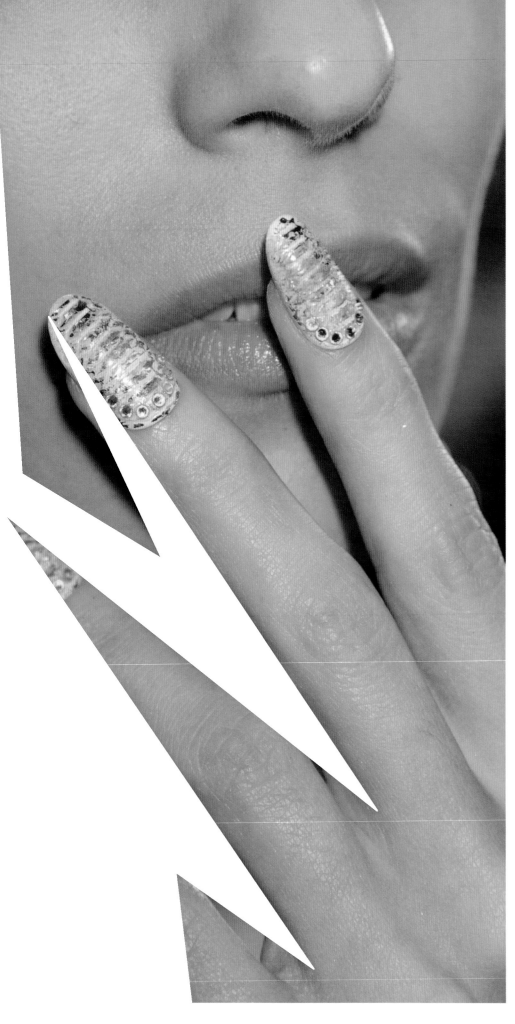

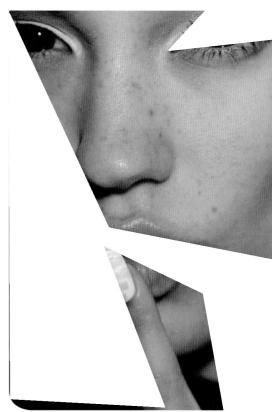

Left *An ombre-style nail look with crystal embellishments and a touch of sparkle by CND for The Blonds Spring/ Summer collection.*

Above *Close-up of a white, textured press-on nail by CND for The Blonds.*

Below *Bright yellow nails with a metallic green layer to add texture by CND for The Blonds.*

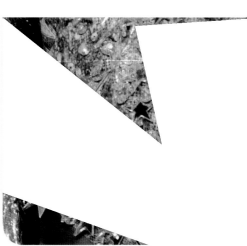

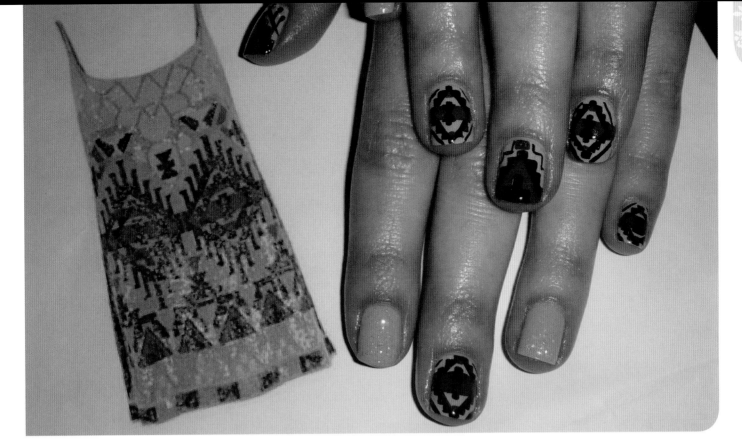

Above *A nail design by Fleury Rose, inspired by the colours, pattern and texture of a dress.*

Fashion Gallery

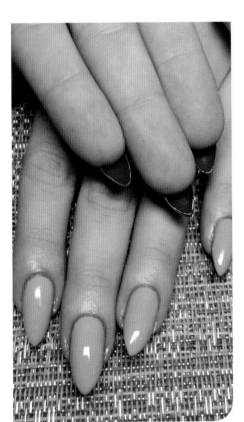

Left *Nails inspired by Christian Louboutin shoes, with a red underside and tip shaped to a point by Fleury Rose.*

Right *A model wears bright pink nail polish applied by Antonio Sacripante to complement the bold colours in fabrics at Stella Jean.*

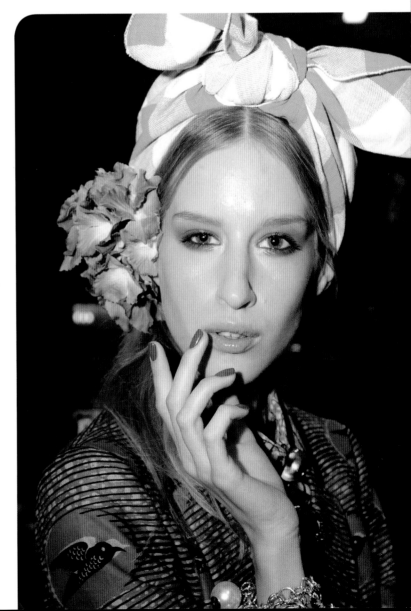

Fashion-forward Fingertips

The advent of nail art on the catwalk is a result of designers recognizing its importance in finishing an overall look and its expression of a personality and trend. A number of designers and key figures in the world of fashion have collaborated with nail brands to produce their own nail collections, based on their seasonal looks or signature styles.

Nail brand Revlon has created appliqués inspired by signature designs from the couture house Marchesa, while the likes of Burberry, Dolce & Gabbana and Tom Ford produce nail-polish shades to coincide with their seasonal collections. The design houses of Giles Deacon and Meadham Kirchoff have lent their names to Nail Rock nail wrap designs and British designer Henry Holland has collaborated with press-on nails from Elegant Touch, so that whatever the budget, catwalk styles can be fashioned by an individual.

Below *Geek-style press-on nails featuring a calculator and glasses, designed by Henry Holland for Elegant Touch.*

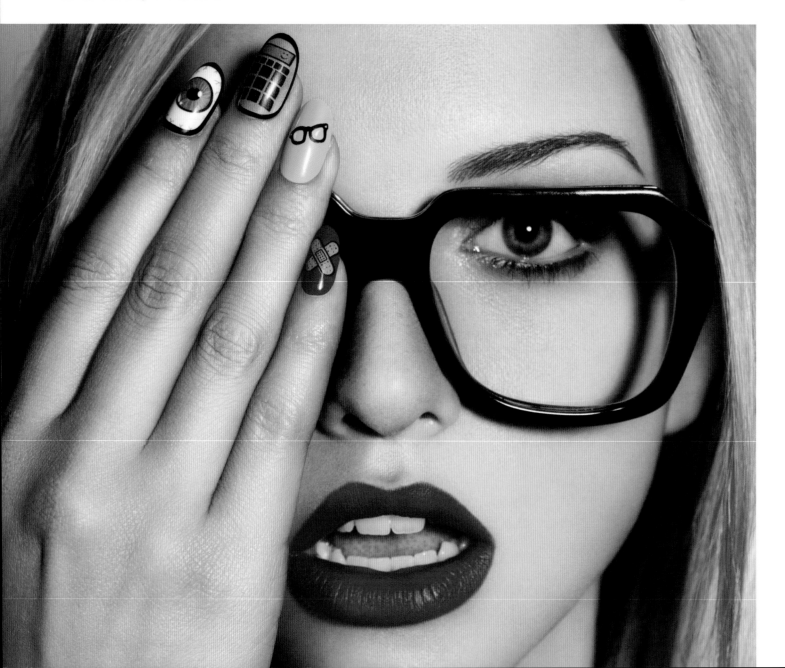

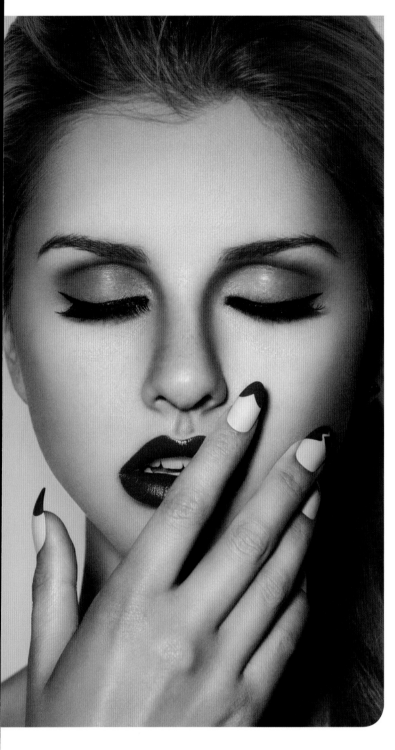

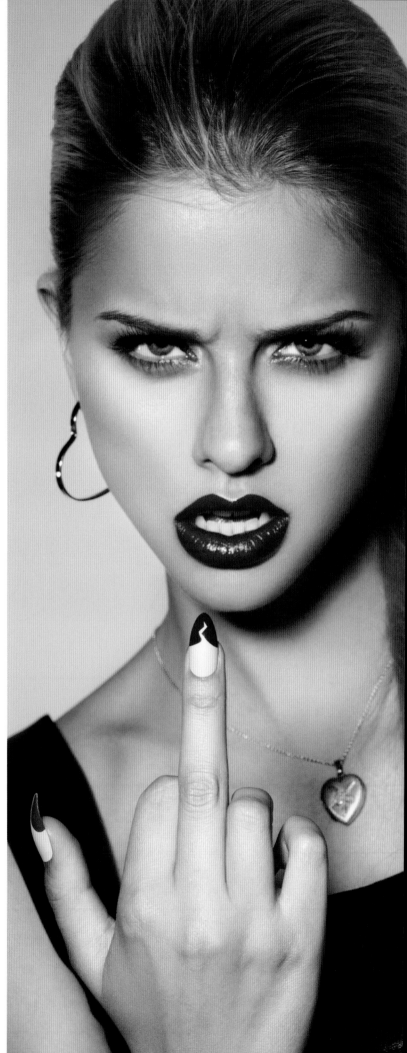

Above *'Heartbreaker' nails – nude with a red heart shape at the tip – designed by Henry Holland for Elegant Touch.*

Right *Almond-shaped nails with a broken heart design by Henry Holland for Elegant Touch.*

STYLE FILE
Henry Holland

British journalism graduate Henry Holland made his foray into the fashion world in 2006 with his 'Fashion Groupies' range of slogan T-shirts, launched under the House of Holland label. The T-shirts, which featured catchphrases incorporating the names of established clothing designers, caught the eye of the fashion world and in February 2008, House of Holland held its first solo show at London Fashion Week.

Henry designs with a 'London Girl' aesthetic in mind and is inspired by the varied attitudes, cultures and mindsets that he sees existing in the British capital. His House of Holland girl is 'cool, confident and savvy and wears labels without letting them wear her'.

Popular with celebrities, House of Holland has lent its design stamp to a number of accessories brands, including hosiery and eyewear. In September 2013, a range of nine press-on nail designs was launched by popular UK nail brand Elegant Touch in collaboration with House of Holland, inspired by his London Fashion Week collections.

'Nails are a statement rather than an afterthought in House of Holland's collections. Finer details such as these are really important when putting together a look. For House of Holland shows, a character is created that is presented as our woman for that season and the finer details are the things that make her; hair, beauty, nails and accessories are all as important as the clothes. Nail art creates, follows and sets trends by itself and is a great, inexpensive way to have fun with fashion and colour.' Henry Holland

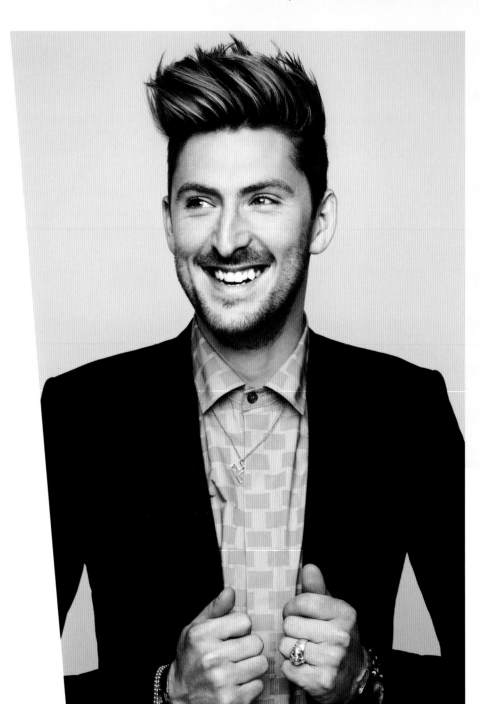

Right *An expressive nail style created using press-on nails from the Henry Holland/Elegant Touch collection.*

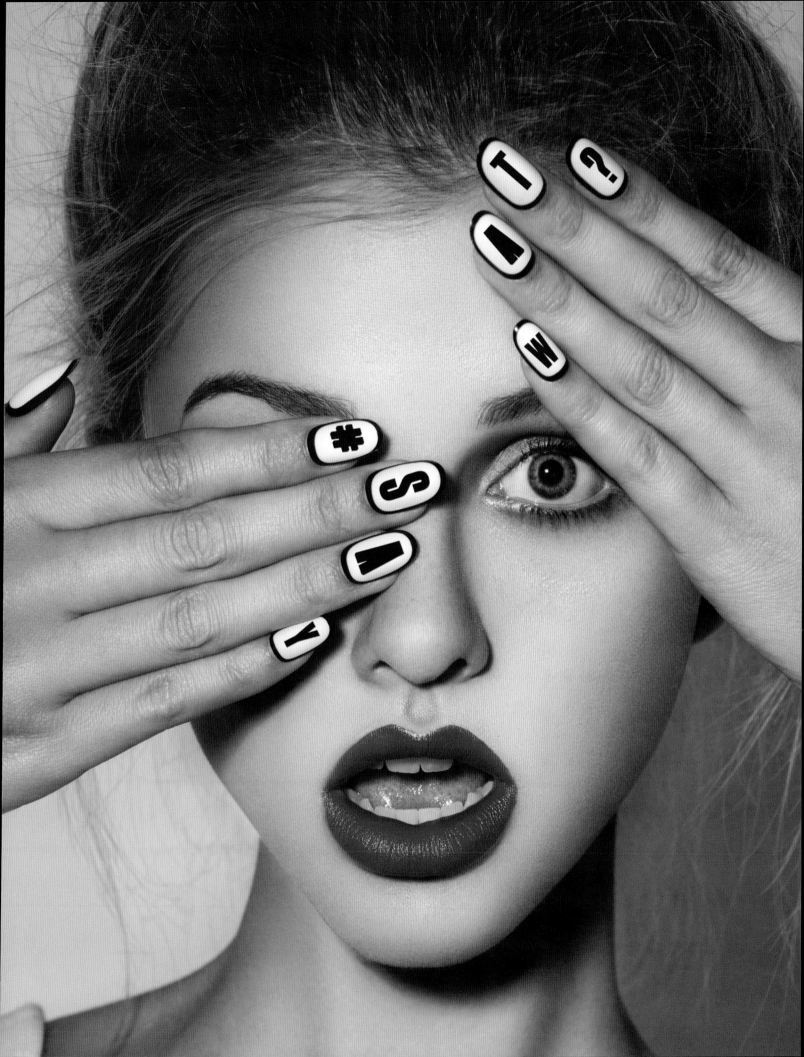

PROJECT: TIGER PRINT by Sam Biddle

Sam Biddle shows how to complement an animal-print fashion item with a nail style for a fashionable finish.

You will need…

1 Base coat

2 Orange glitter polish

3 Water-based acrylic or craft paints in cream, gold and black

4 Thin brush

5 Matte top coat

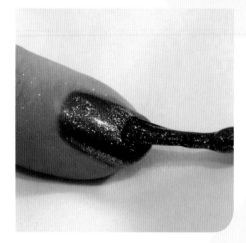

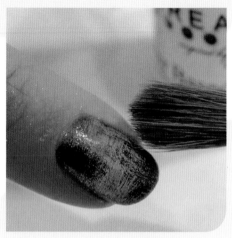

1 Apply a base coat and paint the nails with two thin coats of an orange glitter nail polish. Allow to dry.

2 Use a dry brush, such as an old make-up brush, to brush a cream water-based acrylic paint or craft paint towards the centre of the nail.

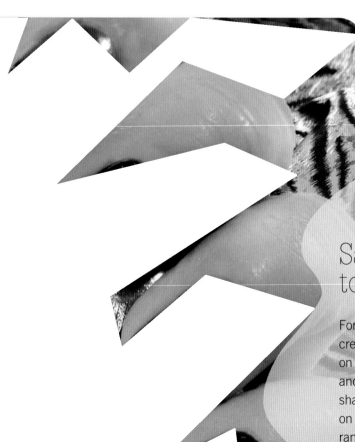

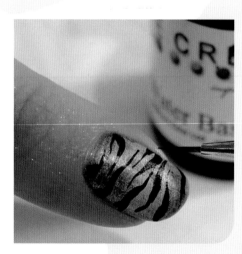

Sam's top tip

For a funkier style, create the tiger stripes on the ring-finger nails and combine the other shades in the project on each nail to create random designs.

4 Use a thin nail-art brush and black nail polish or acrylic paint to paint on tiger stripes with a wide base and tapered point at the end. Work alternately down the nail. Allow to dry.

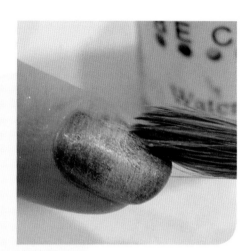

3 Use a gold water-based paint and brush over the cream shade lightly, so all three shades can be seen.

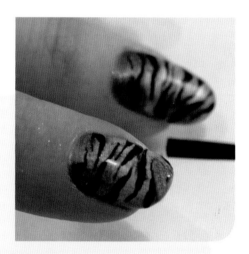

5 Apply a matte top coat to all nails for a softer, more realistic finish.

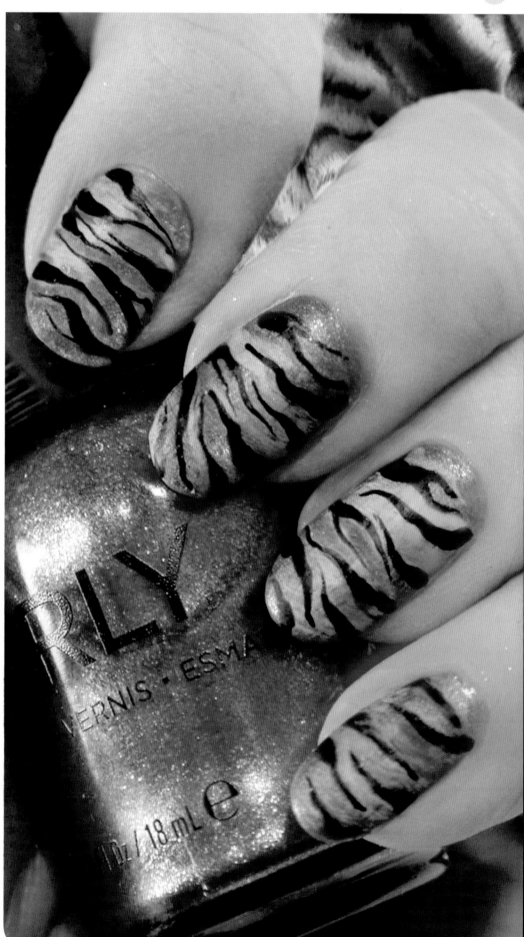

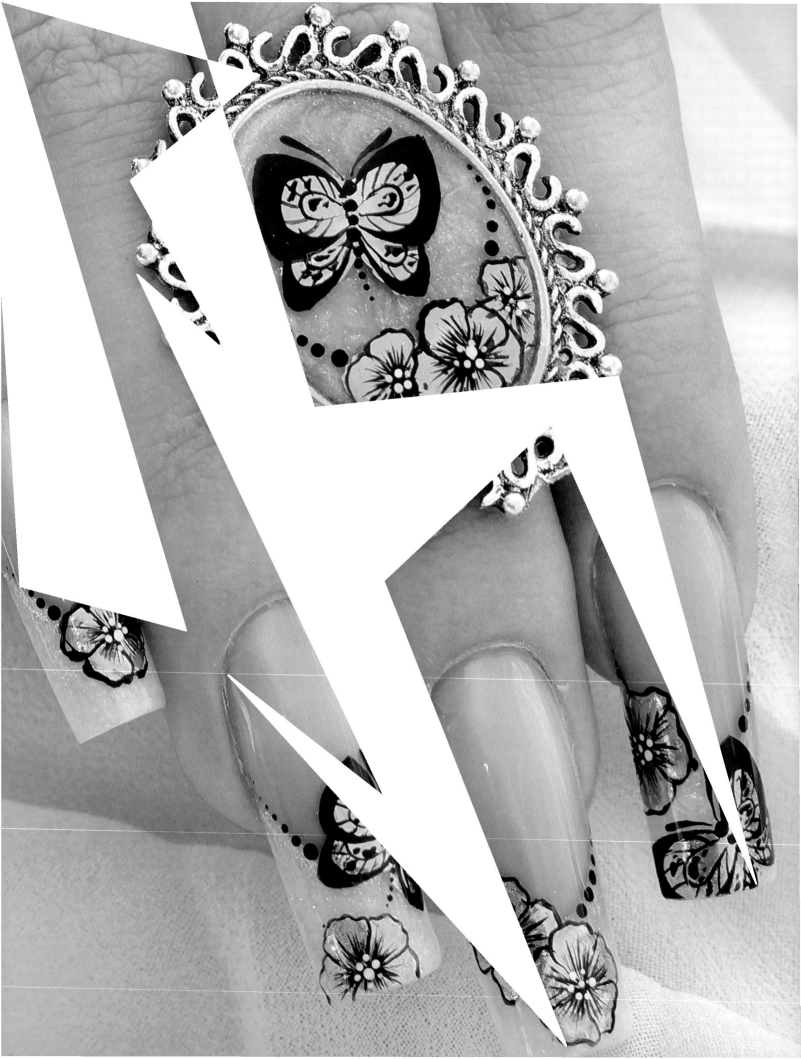

CHAPTER FIVE

ACCESSORIES

A statement necklace, meaningful ring or decorative bag can all influence a nail style, with the accessory and a complementary nail look tying an entire ensemble together. Nail art is often seen as an accessory in itself – a cost-effective way to spruce up an outfit or reflect a trend. The beauty of nail styles is that they can be adapted quickly and easily, serving as an ideal way to pay homage to frequently changing personal accessory choices and clothing fashions.

Accessories form part of daily fashion decisions, reflecting a personal sense of style. The abundance of accessories, from jewellery to bags, scarves, hair items and belts, means that there is a multitude of inspiration for nail styles. Focus on a small area of the accessory and try to replicate that on the nail using polishes, decals and 3D effects to reflect its texture.

The beauty of using an accessory to influence a nail style is that you can adapt the design to your ability. If your nail art skill is limited, take a single element from the accessory such as its colour and then progress to a more detailed replica of the work when skill and time permit.

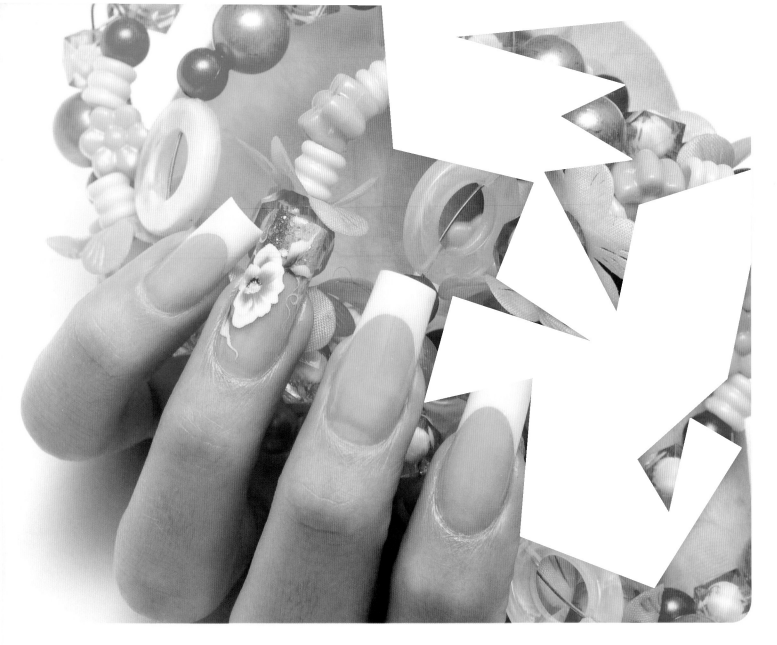

Above *A French manicure with a pretty pink feature nail and floral detailing.*

Right *A hand-painted red floral nail design with a ring to match.*

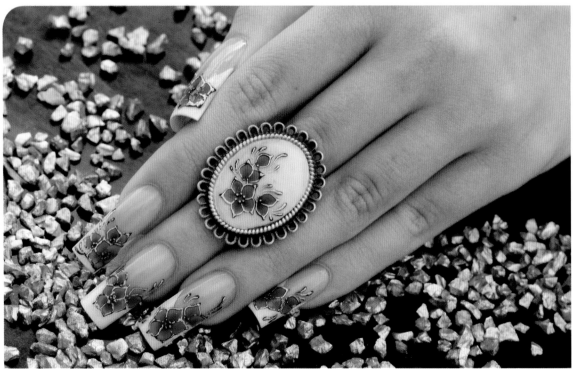

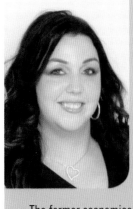

TECHNICIAN PROFILE
Eva Darabos, Hungary

Since entering the nail industry in 2002, Eva Darabos has become well known for her competition success, attaining 12 gold medals at the renowned Nailympia London using a variety of nail-styling techniques and products.

The former economics graduate holds the titles of three times European nail champion and 12 times Hungary's national champion. She travels all over the world sharing her expertise with fellow nail technicians as well as running a salon in Budapest, where she founded the Eva Darabos Nail Academy to train up-and-coming nail technicians in product application and design.

Below *An unusual nail shape featuring shades of turquoise and white to match the accessory.*

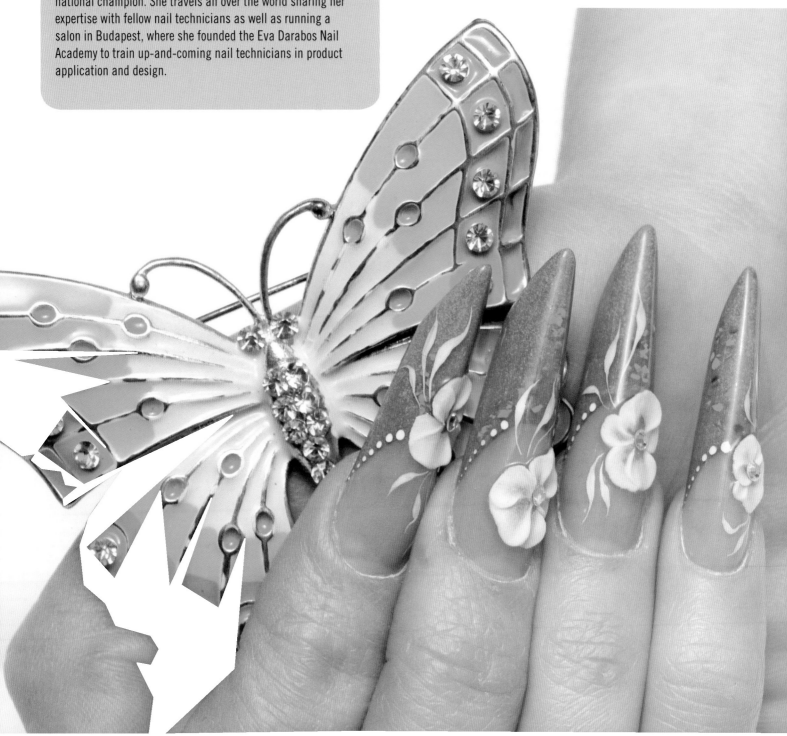

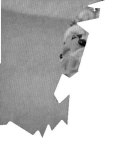

Ideas to Accessorize

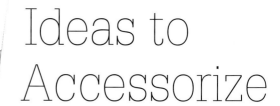

To find inspiration for a wide range of nail designs, regard all objects as accessories, from sweet wrappers to playing cards and items from themed occasions. The objects can even be used within the design itself; flat objects such as wrappers can be cut and secured to the nail plate with nail glue if freehand nail art proves tricky or there is limited time.

Taking advantage of texture can also help to complement an item. Sprinkle small beads over a wet top coat and allow to dry for a 3D effect to match jewellery, or opt for special effects polishes, such as those that leave a leather or denim-like finish, to match nails to a bag or item of clothing.

Above *Elegant stiletto nails by Michelle Sproat, created to complement an evening bag.*

Below *Megumi Mizuno found inspiration from a pack of cards to create a 3D design on nail tips.*

Opposite top left *Black, matte nails with studded embellishments by Sophie Harris-Greenslade.*

Opposite top right *A 3D nail design by Sophie Harris-Greenslade inspired by a Fabergé egg, featuring polish, gold nail foils and an assortment of beads.*

Right *Hand-painted designs on nail tips by Sam Biddle, inspired by confectionery.*

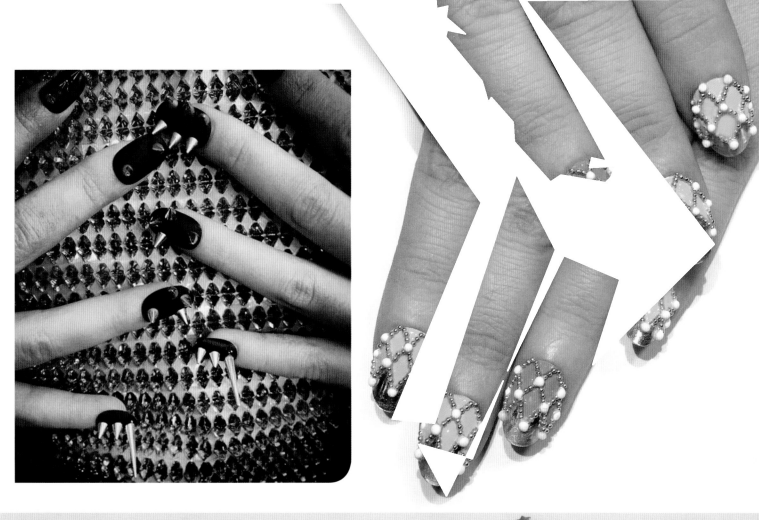

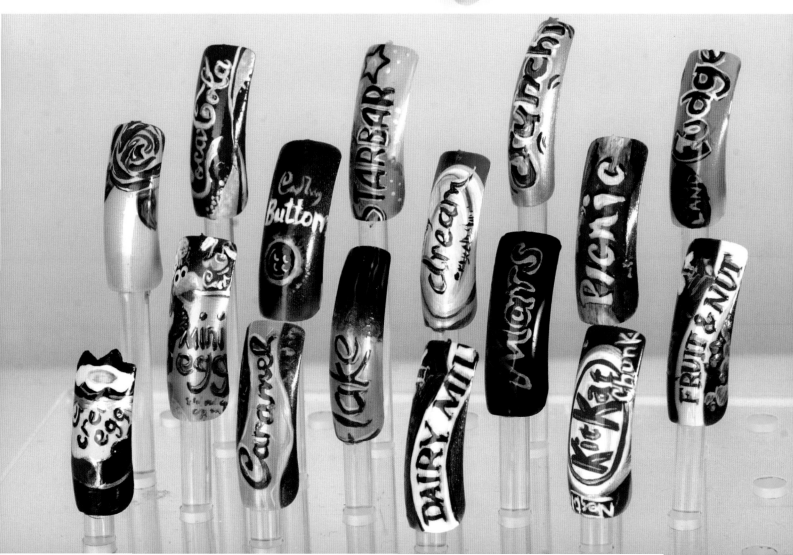

PROJECT: ACCESSORY-INSPIRED NAILS by Eva Darabos

Eva Darabos shows how to complement statement jewellery items with a chic nail design.

You will need

1 Base coat

2 Silver metallic nail polish

3 Black nail polish

4 Thin brush

5 Crystals or diamantés

6 Top coat

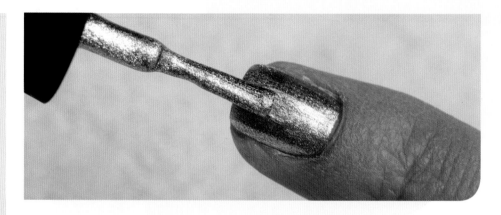

1 Apply base coat followed by two thin layers of a silver metallic nail polish on all the nails except those on the ring fingers.

2 Apply base coat followed by two thin coats of black nail polish to the ring-finger nails. Allow to dry for at least two minutes.

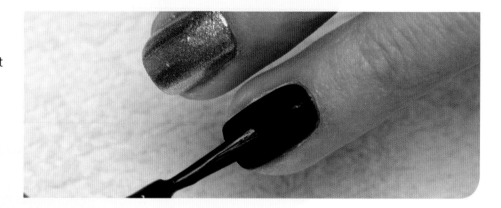

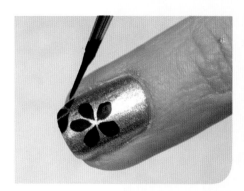

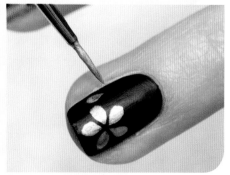

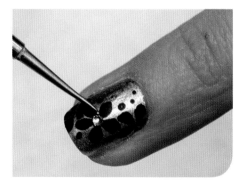

3 Dip a thin brush with a pointed end into the black nail polish and create flower designs on each of the silver nails. Change the position, size and number of flowers across these eight nails.

4 Repeat step 3 on the ring-finger nails but this time use the silver nail polish instead.

5 Complete each nail design by adding some dots around the flowers. Add a dab of top coat into the centre of some of the flowers and affix a crystal or diamanté. Allow the design to dry.

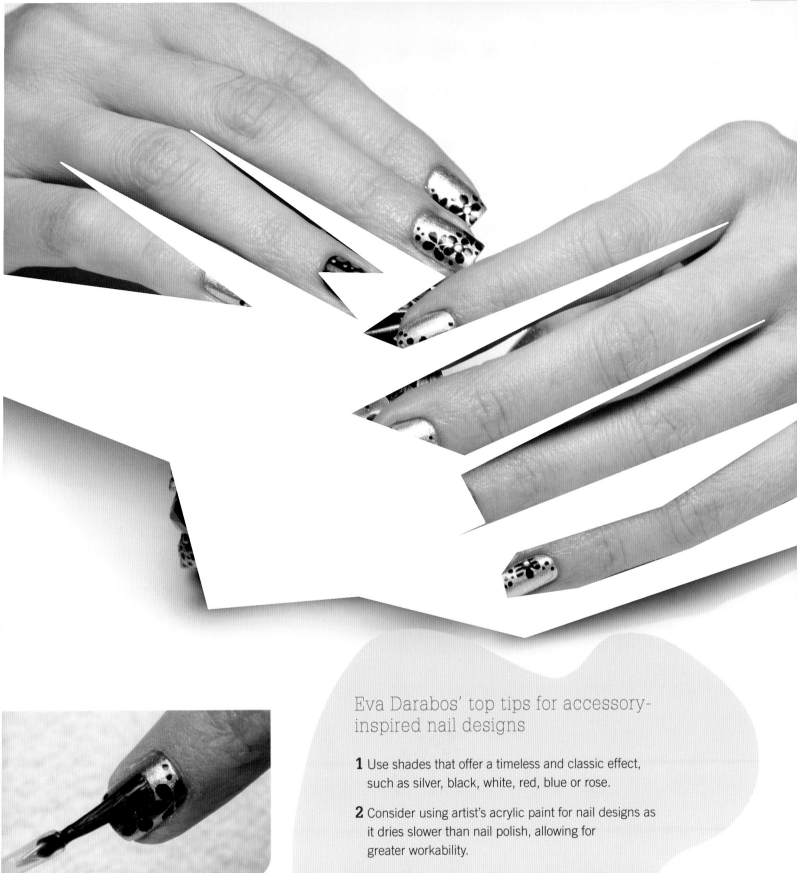

6 Apply a thin layer of top coat to all the nails and allow to dry.

Eva Darabos' top tips for accessory-inspired nail designs

1 Use shades that offer a timeless and classic effect, such as silver, black, white, red, blue or rose.

2 Consider using artist's acrylic paint for nail designs as it dries slower than nail polish, allowing for greater workability.

3 Experiment with top coats such as matte, glitter, glossy or holographic for a super-eye-catching nail finish.

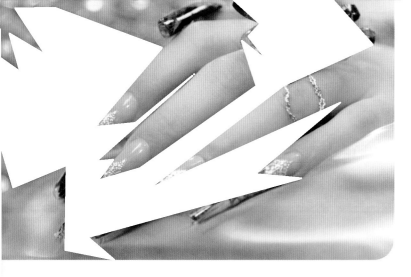

Image Gallery

Left *A pretty ring with nails to complement it, designed by Catherine Wong and featuring encapsulated foil and hand-painted silver details.*

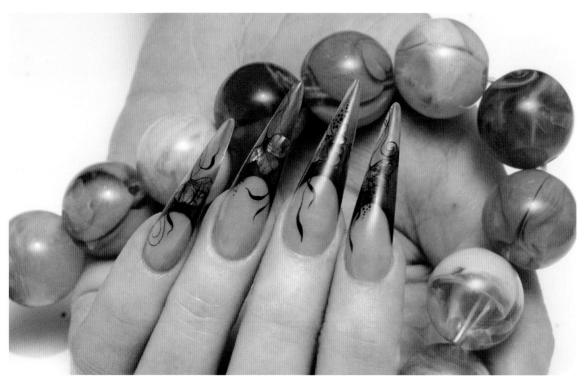

Left *Nails inspired by beads in both colour and form, by Eva Darabos.*

Bottom *Extended nails with dotted detailing at the smile line and hues of blue at the tip, by Eva Darabos.*

Right *Sparkly nails by Fleury Rose featuring flowers and details, inspired by a ring.*

Far right *Dazzling oval-shaped nails in jewel tones and embellished with crystals by Sophie Harris-Greenslade, designed to complement jewellery.*

Bottom right *Sophisticated, short black nails by Sophie Harris-Greenslade, with gold foil details to complement the rings.*

Bottom far right *A colourful nail design by Sam Biddle featuring shades and sparkle inspired by the accessory.*

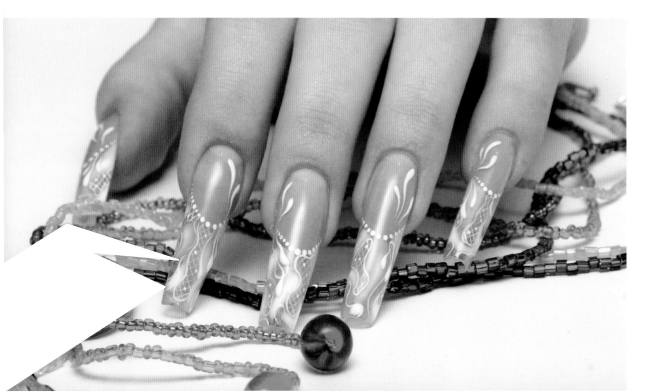

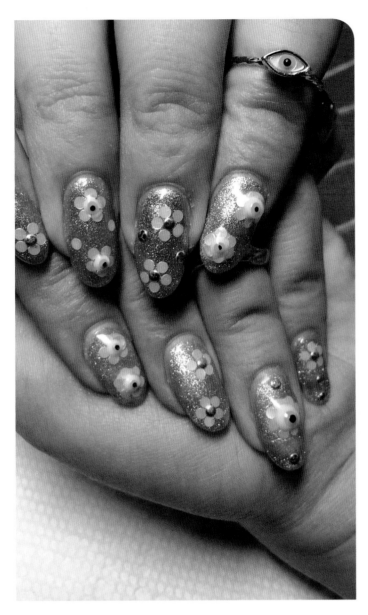
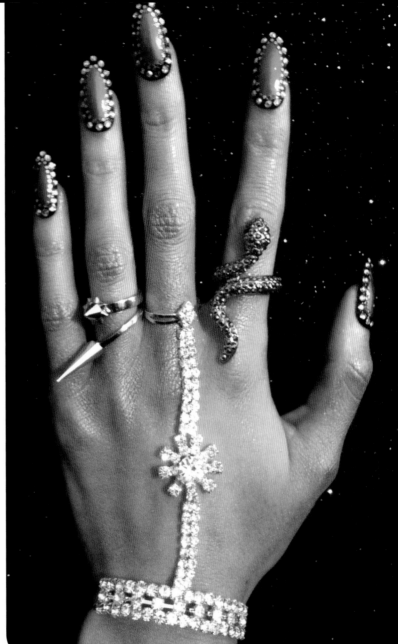
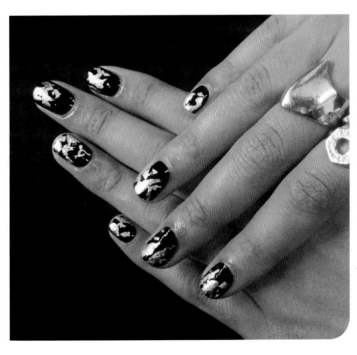
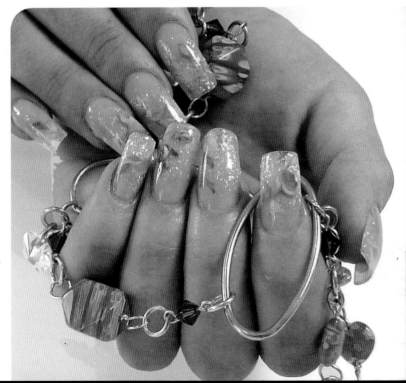

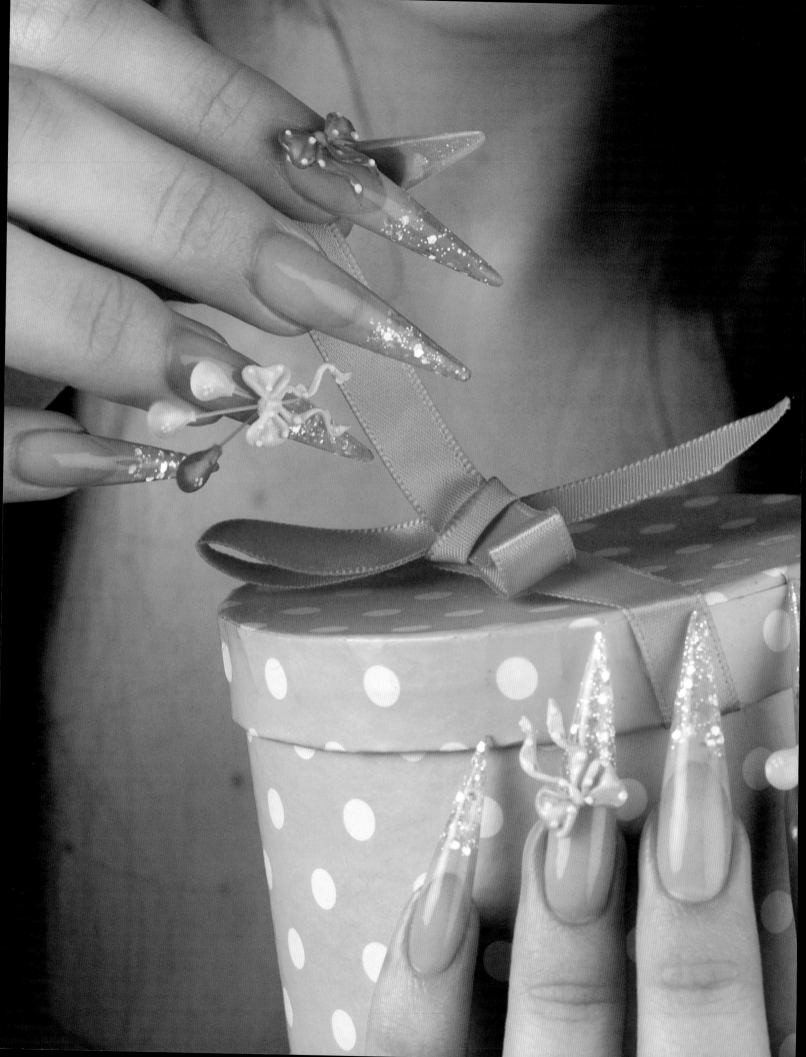

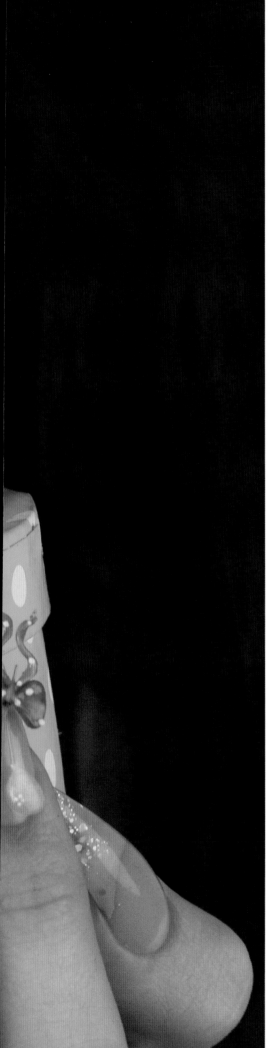

CHAPTER SIX

NAILS FOR SPECIAL EVENTS

Nails fit for a special occasion or periodic event can be a fun way to get into the spirit of the moment, and the possibilities for design are numerous; use a calendar to note the events coming up so you have plenty of time to determine your nail style of choice. If the occasion is a short affair such as a birthday, awards event or Valentine's Day, nail polish is ideal, whereas for longer events such as the Christmas season, enhancements will mean the nail art design will last for up to three weeks.

With special occasion nails, the design can be as simple or as complex as desired, dependent on the nail technician. For a subtle nod to the event, consider a feature nail design in relevant colours, or for an eye-catching design, ask your technician for decals, an unusual nail shape or sculpted 3D art. There are no rules with regard to special-occasion nails, but look to the associated objects and colours for inspiration.

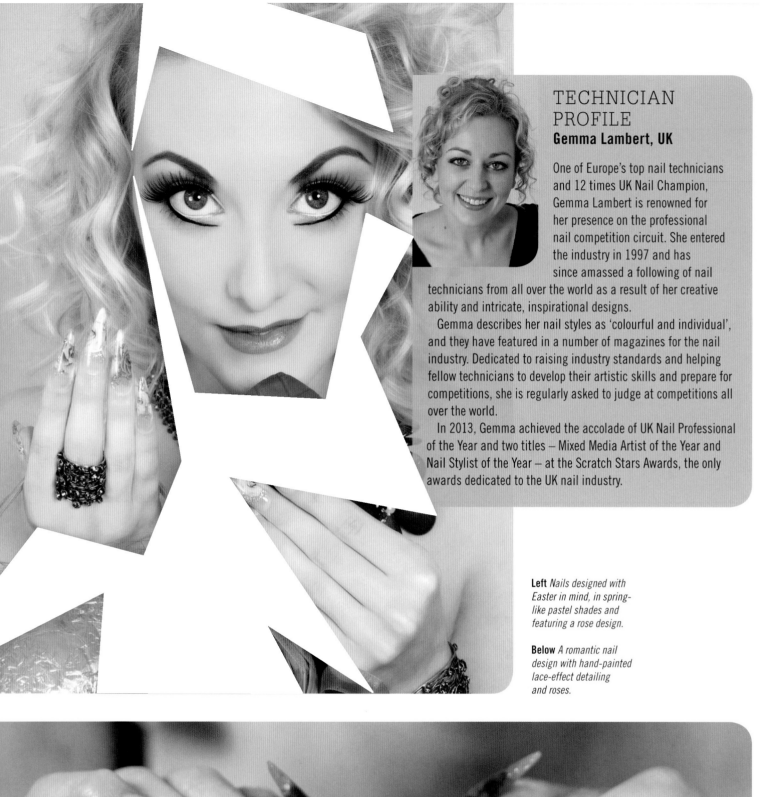

TECHNICIAN PROFILE
Gemma Lambert, UK

One of Europe's top nail technicians and 12 times UK Nail Champion, Gemma Lambert is renowned for her presence on the professional nail competition circuit. She entered the industry in 1997 and has since amassed a following of nail technicians from all over the world as a result of her creative ability and intricate, inspirational designs.

Gemma describes her nail styles as 'colourful and individual', and they have featured in a number of magazines for the nail industry. Dedicated to raising industry standards and helping fellow technicians to develop their artistic skills and prepare for competitions, she is regularly asked to judge at competitions all over the world.

In 2013, Gemma achieved the accolade of UK Nail Professional of the Year and two titles — Mixed Media Artist of the Year and Nail Stylist of the Year — at the Scratch Stars Awards, the only awards dedicated to the UK nail industry.

Left *Nails designed with Easter in mind, in spring-like pastel shades and featuring a rose design.*

Below *A romantic nail design with hand-painted lace-effect detailing and roses.*

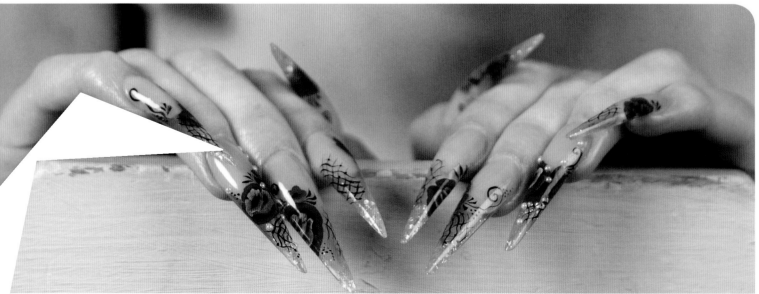

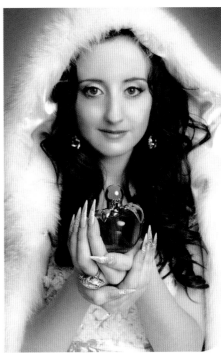

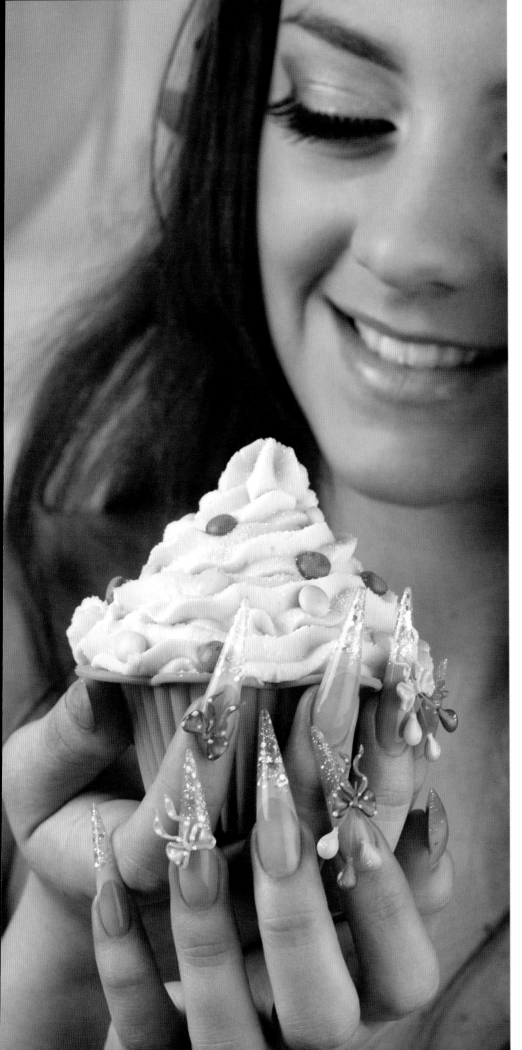

Above *Nails inspired by Snow White in a pale shade with glitter embellishments.*

Left *Celebratory nails sculpted to a stiletto shape with 3D design elements.*

Left *Stiletto shape nails inspired by the Queen of Hearts with hand-painted lace and rose detail.*

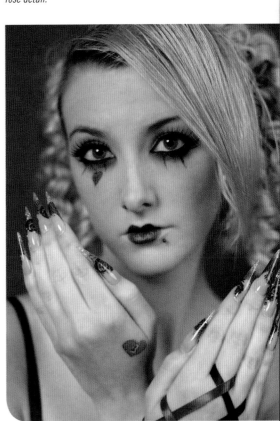

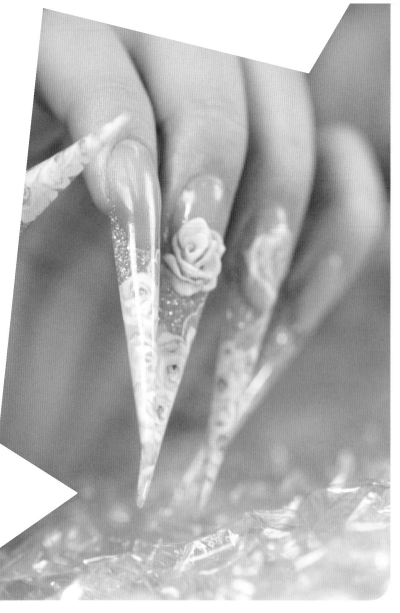

Bridal Style

A wedding day is expected to be one of the most important days of all, when a couple are joined in unity and love. All eyes and cameras will be on the bride and groom, and as they show off their wedding rings their hands and nails become a key focus. Nails speak volumes about a person, indicating their lifestyle as well as their personal sense of style, so a groom should ensure clean, well-shaped and short nails for the wedding day. The bride, on the other hand, can choose from a large range of nail styles, based on a number of ideas and influences.

The French manicure is always a popular choice for a traditional bride. Enhancing the appearance of the natural nail, with its pink nail bed and white tip, a French manicure offers a well-groomed and subtle look that doesn't distract attention from the bride or her dress. However, with pops of colour, varying fabrics and multiple accessories often present at a wedding, from the bride and bridesmaid's dresses to flowers and table settings, the bride may choose to

Left *A sparkly stiletto-shaped nail design by Catherine Wong, with hand-painted white roses and a sculpted rose design on the feature nail.*

Below left *French-style nails by Sam Biddle with a chevron shape and a touch of something blue.*

Below *An extravagant bridal nail style by Sam Biddle, featuring 3D sculpted flowers possibly designed with the bride's bouquet in mind.*

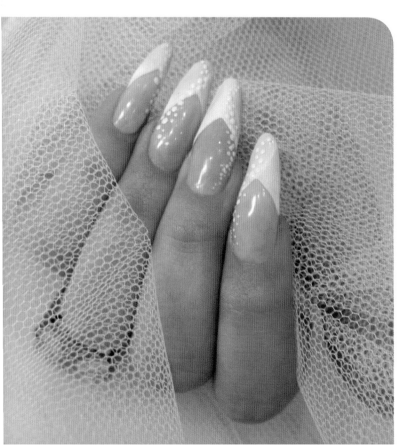

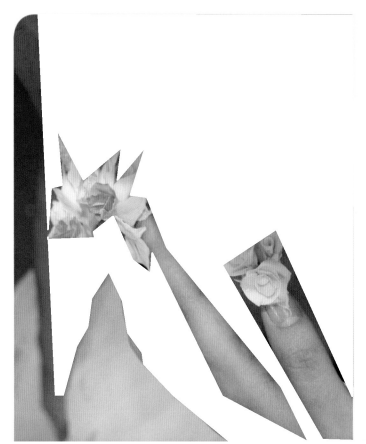

incorporate these elements in her nail design to encompass the overall style of the day.

Many nail technicians can sculpt designs such as flowers on top of the nail for a 3D effect or take one of the wedding fabrics and either encapsulate it within the nail or re-create it using a freehand technique. The complexity of the design is entirely up to the bride and the capabilities of her nail technician, who will usually create a design a day or two before the big day, or on the day if just using nail polish on the bride's natural nails. Depending on her footwear, a bride's toenails are often painted in a French manicure design or a shade appropriate for her honeymoon.

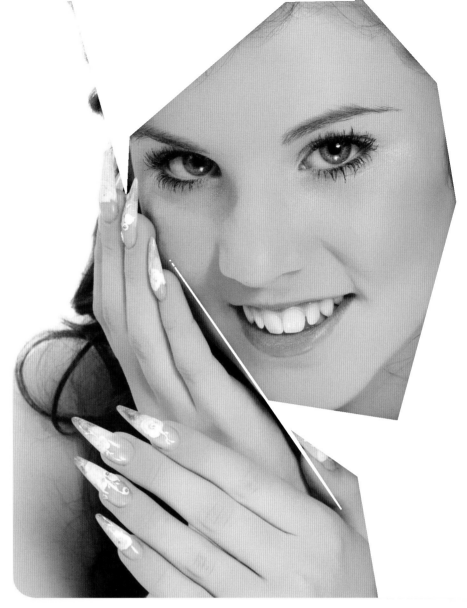

Right *A feminine nail shape with white floral detailing and crystal embellishments by Gemma Lambert.*

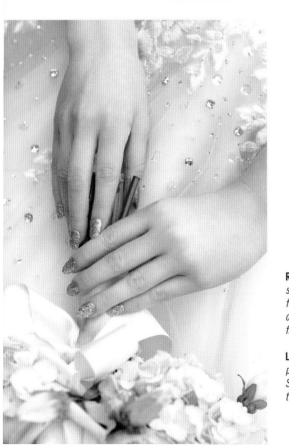

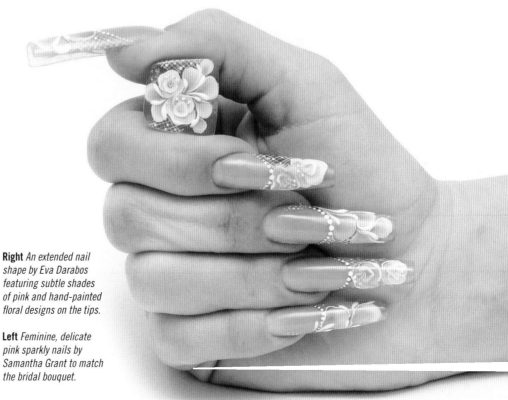

Right *An extended nail shape by Eva Darabos featuring subtle shades of pink and hand-painted floral designs on the tips.*

Left *Feminine, delicate pink sparkly nails by Samantha Grant to match the bridal bouquet.*

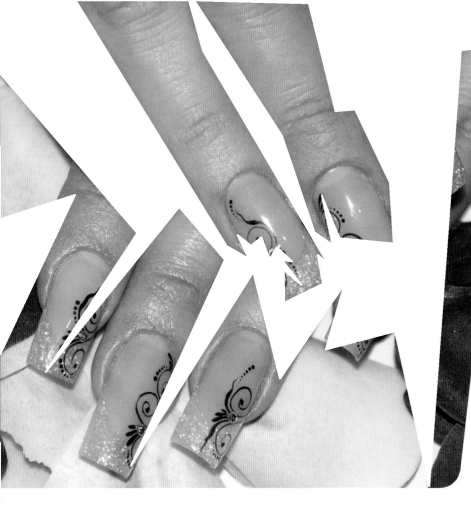

Shape

Long nails exude elegance and femininity, and the stiletto nail shape, while not the most practical if you are not used to the length, can be a great choice. Nail technicians can craft this shape with professional nail products and embed colours, decals and designs within it according to your theme.

Shorter, almond-shaped or square nails are more practical, and professional enhancements can extend the shape beyond the natural nail. A curved tip allows a design to be seen from a number of angles – ideal when guests are taking photographs from varied positions.

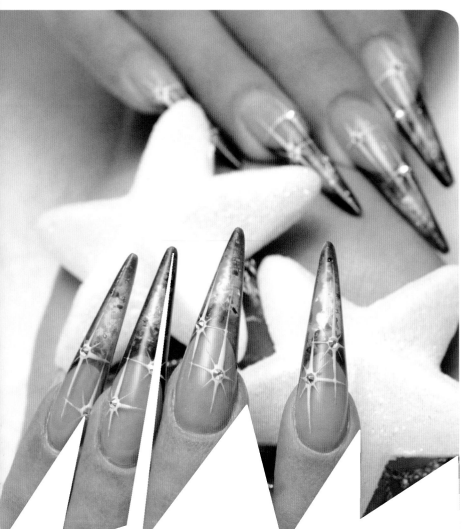

Above left *Extended, square nails with glitter tips and hand-painted details by Eva Darabos.*

Left *Stiletto-shaped nail enhancements by Eva Darabos, featuring an eye-catching turquoise shade, glitter and embellishments.*

Below *Short white nails with a festive red glitter effect reminiscent of a candy cane, by Sam Biddle.*

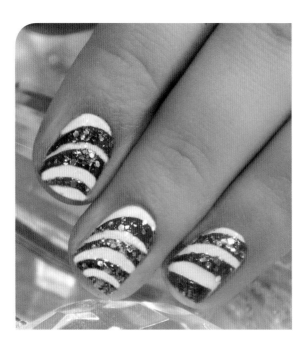

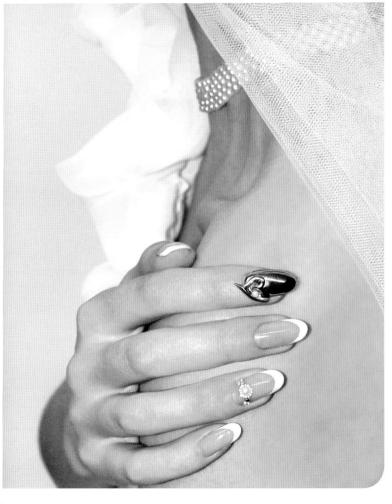

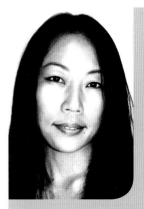

TECHNICIAN PROFILE
Megumi Mizuno, Japan

Before commencing her career as an international award-winning nail artist, Megumi Mizuno already had artistic experiences in a host of creative arenas which she could draw on for technique and inspiration. From an early age, Megumi would often be found drawing or painting and it was not long before her grandmother, a professional watercolour painter, spotted her natural talent and a private tutor was employed to nurture it. Once at university, Megumi studied Environmental Design, which encompassed urban development design and landscape design. This was followed by further study, in subjects including Auto CAD, Photoshop and web design. It was in between her studies and various jobs that Megumi started to explore her interest in nail art for personal use. Her curiosity about this medium culminated in her attaining VTCT Levels 2 and 3 at Redbridge College in Romford, UK, setting her upon her current career path.

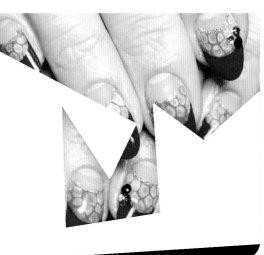

Above *An unusual twist on the classic French manicure, with a chrome index-finger nail and embellishments on the ring finger.*

Left *A striking take on the half-moon manicure, with a snakeskin-style print and scarlet nail tips.*

Right *Bold, bright and fun nails in a random design.*

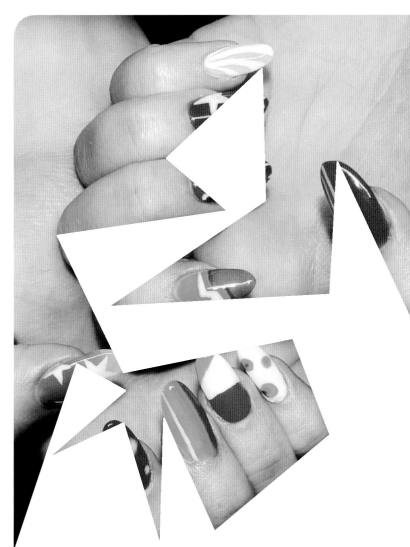

Awards

Finalist - Scratch Stars Awards Mixed Media Artist of the Year 2013 & 2014

Finalist - Scratch Stars Awards Nail Artist of the Year 2012

Finalist - Scratch Stars Awards Gel Polish Stylist of the Year 2012 & 2014

2nd (Division 3) - Mixed Media Master - Nailympia London 2012

1st - Showcase Nail Art - Professional Beauty Manchester 2011

2nd - Showcase Nail Art - London International Nail Competition 2011

1st - The Nail Team's Photographic Competition 2010

1st - Top Tech Boxed Art - Beauty UK 2010

Image Gallery

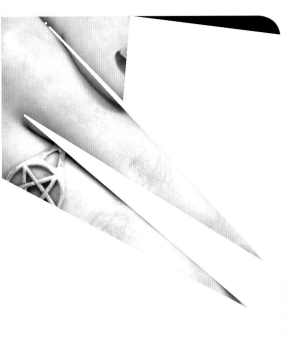

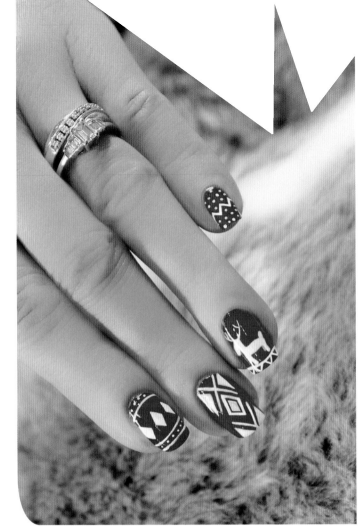

Left *Halloween-style nails by Sam Biddle in appropriate shades of black and orange, with hand-painted details.*

Right *Red nails with Christmassy nail art painted in white by Sam Biddle.*

Below right *Oval nails with a hand-painted heart design by Sophie Harris-Greenslade.*

Below left *British-themed nails in a scarlet shade by Sam Biddle, with a hand-painted Union Jack on the ring finger.*

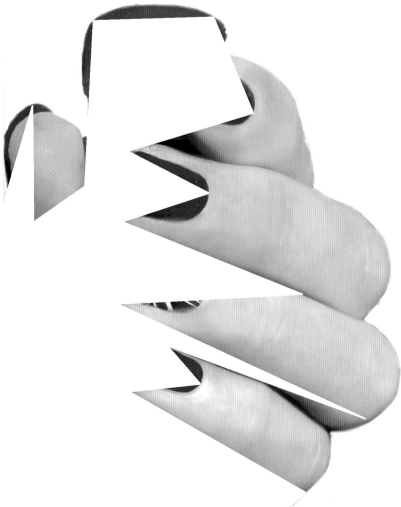

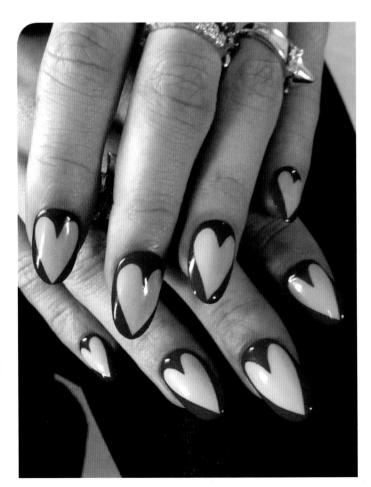

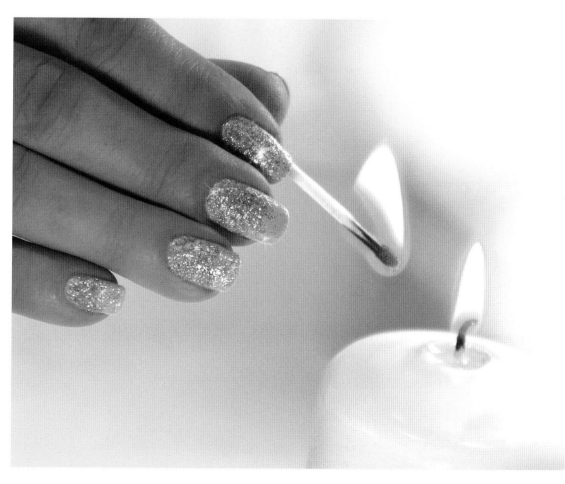

Left *A gold glitter manicure fit for any occasion by Sam Biddle.*

Below *Disco-style holographic nails by Sophie Harris-Greenslade.*

Below left *Nail art inspired by Christmas knitwear, painted freehand in festive shades of red, blue and white by Sophie Harris-Greenslade.*

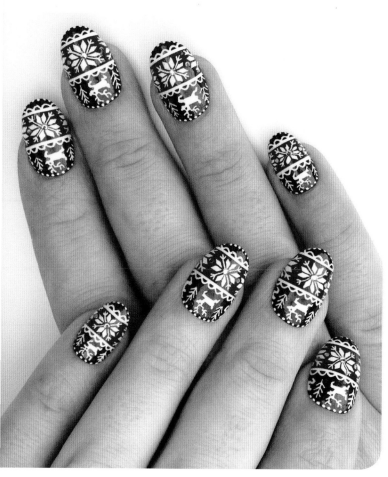

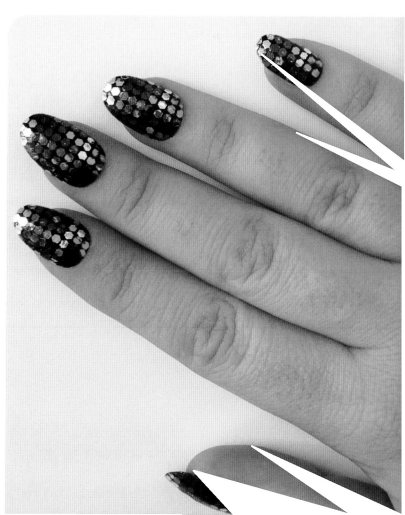

PROJECT: RED VELVET LOVE HEARTS by Sam Biddle

Showing a subtle way to acknowledge Valentine's Day, Sam Biddle
creates a design featuring a statement nail, adding a textured
element to the manicure.

You will need

1 Base coat

2 Nude or pale pink polish

3 Thin brush

4 White, red and black nail
   polishes

5 Buffer

6 Top coat

7 Pencil

8 Red velvet dustings

9 Fantail brush

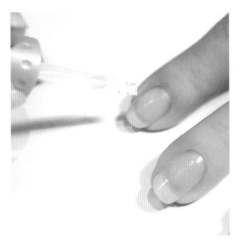

1 Apply a base coat to the nails,
followed by one coat of nude or
pale pink polish on all the nails except
those on the ring fingers.

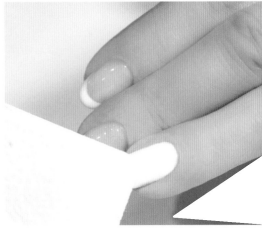

2 With a thin brush and white
polish, create a white tip on the
nails in French manicure style. On the
ring fingers, apply two coats of white
polish then apply top coat to all the
nails. When the ring fingers are dry,
lightly buff the surface of these nails
only to create a matte finish.

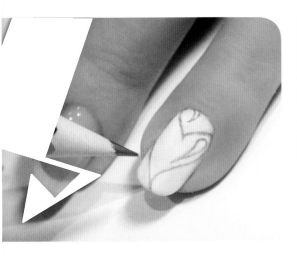

3 Draw a heart design on the white
polish using pencil. The pencil
marks can be erased if you make
any mistakes.

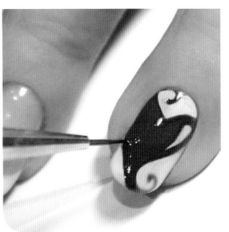

4 Dip a thin brush in red polish and
fill in the heart shape.

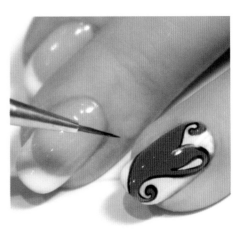

5 Enhance the shape by outlining
it using a black water-based nail
paint or polish.

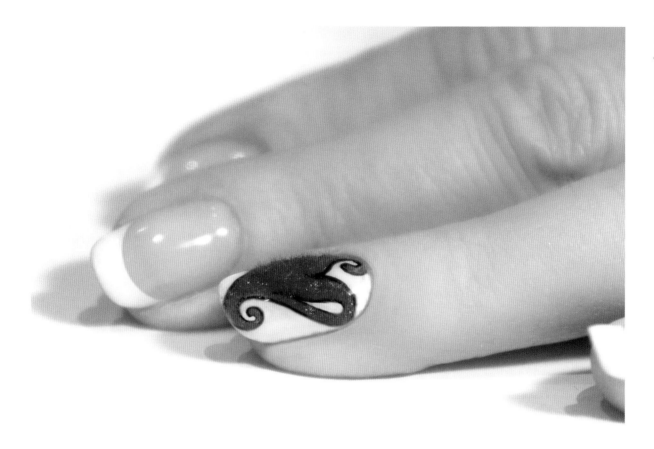

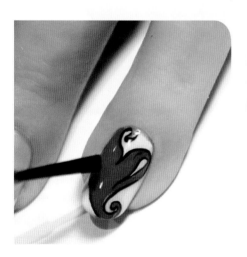

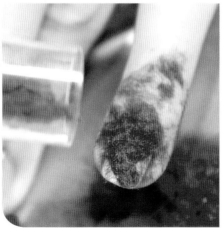

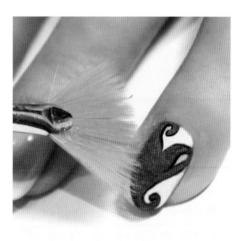

6 Allow the nails to dry fully and apply a layer of clear top coat to all of them.

7 When the ring-finger nails are dry, use a brush to apply another layer of top coat to the heart shape only. Sprinkle red velvet over the top coat on these nails while wet.

8 Leave to dry for 30 seconds before removing any excess velvet with a small brush.

PROJECT: BIRTHDAY BALLOON NAILS by Gemma Lambert

Create a balloon design on nails for a fun, eye-catching
way to acknowledge an occasion or celebration. Gemma
Lambert shows how.

You will need

1 Base coat

2 White nail polish

3 Your choice of six bright shades
of nail polish

4 Black nail polish or striper

5 A thin nail art brush and
dotting tool

6 Top coat

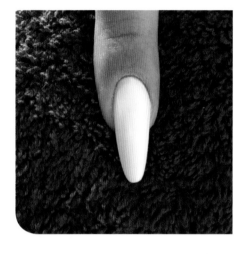

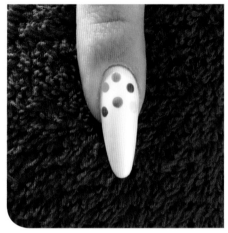

1 Shape nails to a point and apply base coat, followed by two coats of an opaque white nail polish.

2 Using a dotting tool and an assortment of nail polish shades, add dots towards the cuticle end of the nail, allowing space in between them.

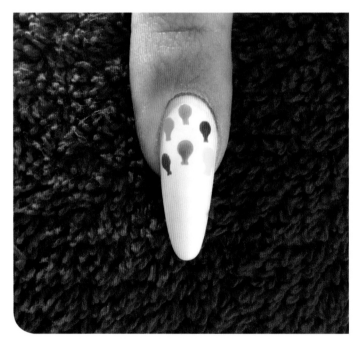

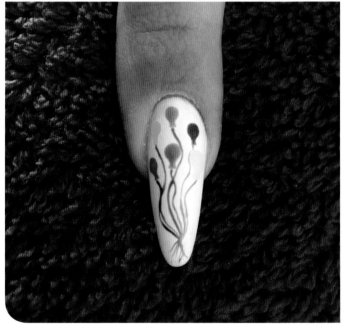

3 Use a thin brush or the smaller end of the dotting tool to extend the shape in the direction of the free edge of the nail to create the base of the balloon.

4 With black nail polish and a thin brush or a black nail striper, create the balloon ribbons, heading in a swirly shape towards the end of the nail.

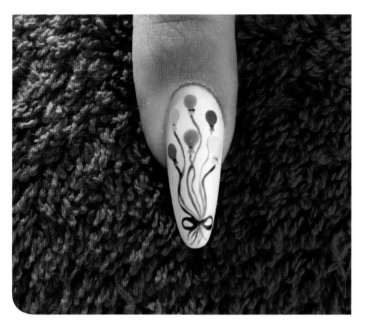

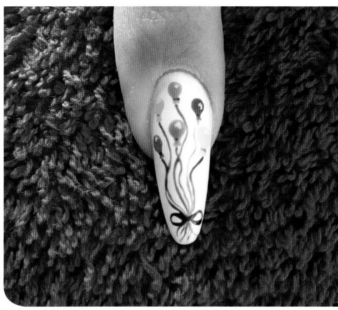

5 Add a bow to tie the painted ribbons together, and add dashes of black polish towards the end of the balloons to create the tied effect.

6 Use a thin brush and white nail polish to add a shine-effect detail to the balloons. Allow to dry and seal with a thin layer of top coat.

More birthday nails...

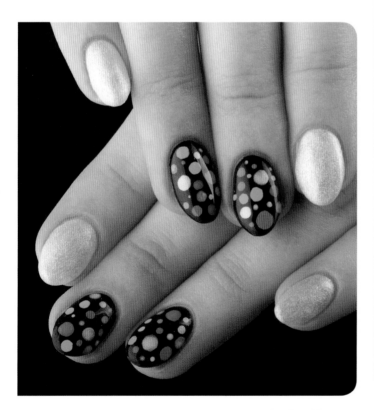

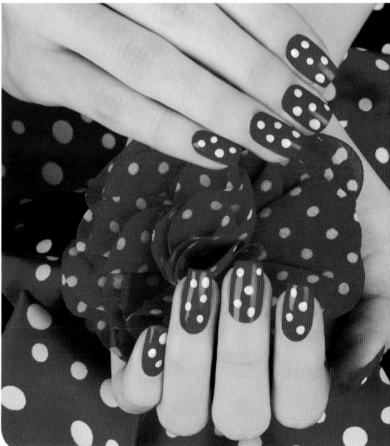

For simple and eye catching occasion nails, try out this great multi-coloured dot design, to compliment the black base and neon dots use a light sparkle polish on the remaining nails.

Bright, fun and very easy to achieve. You could use any base colour of your choice for these polka dot nails.

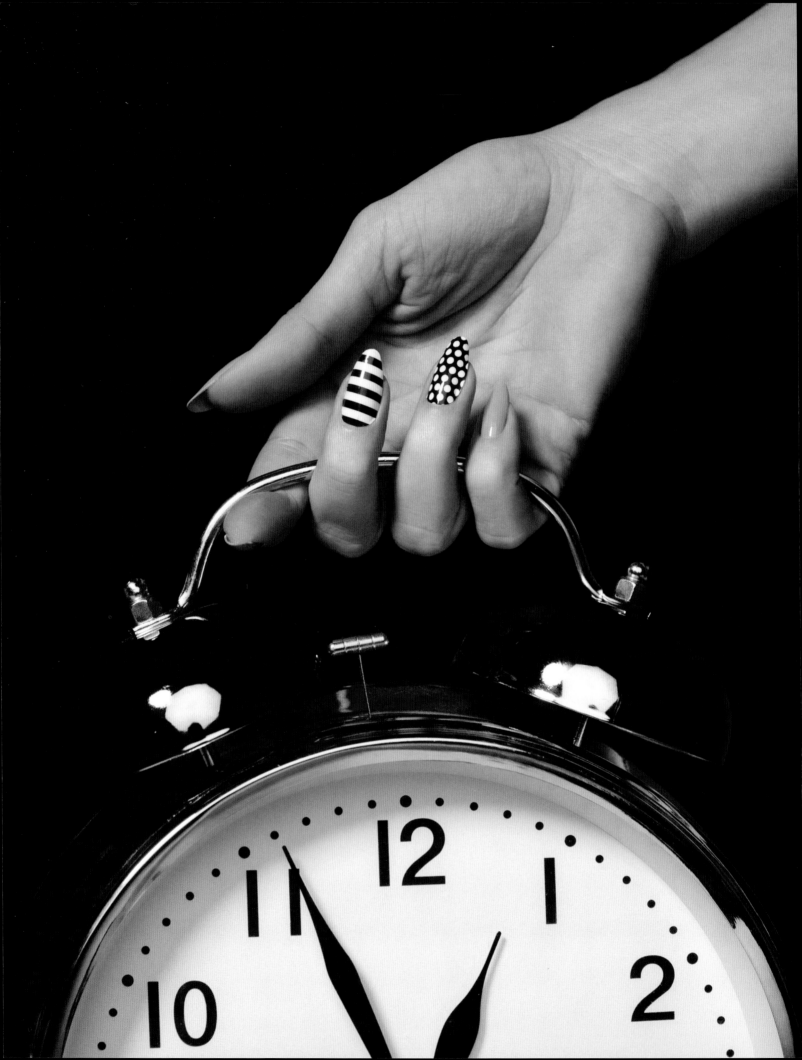

CHAPTER SEVEN

LOOKING TO THE PAST

History books and other research materials can generate inspiration for nail artistry, providing information on popular shades, shapes and patterns from past eras so that whether it was hundreds of years or just several decades ago, appreciation for the era can be expressed in a modern format.

For quick-fix nail styles, nail stickers or wraps are a good option, while if a more intricate and long-lasting design is wanted, and there is time to spare, a professional nail enhancement with sculpted or encapsulated features and custom freehand work can be created by a nail technician.

Left *Randomly patterned nails by Beth Fricke, featuring monochrome designs and a striking turquoise crème shade.*

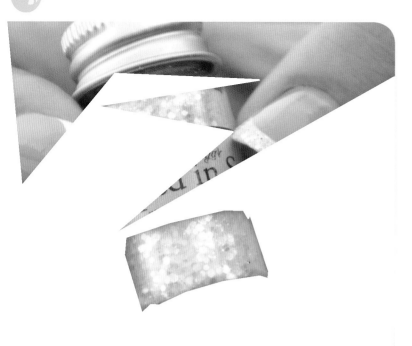

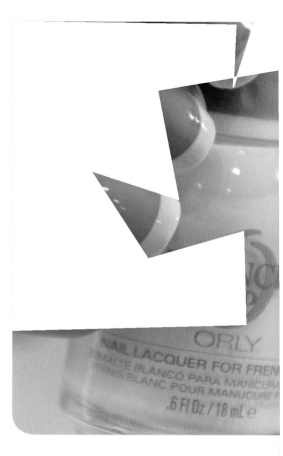

Left *A French manicure with sparkling tip.*

Right *The classic French manicure using nail lacquer.*

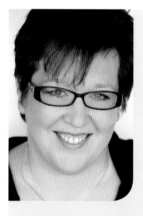

TECHNICIAN PROFILE
Sam Biddle, UK

International nail judge and competition-winner Sam Biddle has found global success with her renowned design and colour skills. Since her first foray into the nail industry in 2000 she has produced front covers for magazines in Europe and the USA, opened her own salon and nail academy and founded Be Inspired, a company that produces a series of nail art tools and products to help nail art fans achieve the designs they desire.

As an independent global educator, Sam teaches new and advanced skills to nail technicians and works with various distributors and product houses internationally, developing brands and providing training. She regularly contributes to trade and consumer press and believes that through the power of creativity, and from the inspiration all around, anyone can achieve the highest flights in nail style.

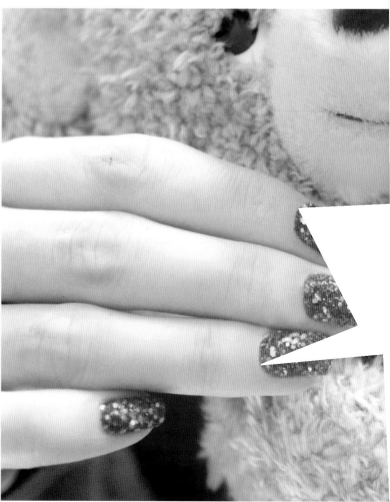

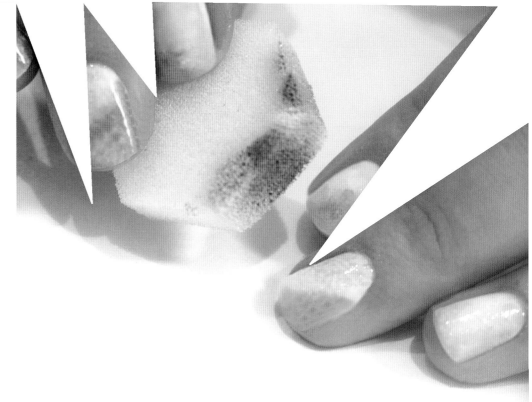

Below *The 'dipped in sugar' effect combines varying sizes of glitter for a holographic bling finish.*

Right *Colourful gradient nails created using a sponge and nail lacquer.*

Below right *Hand-painted blue and white nails in comic-book style.*

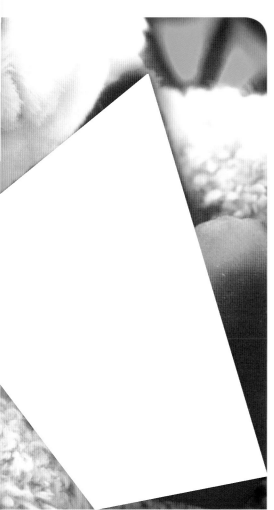

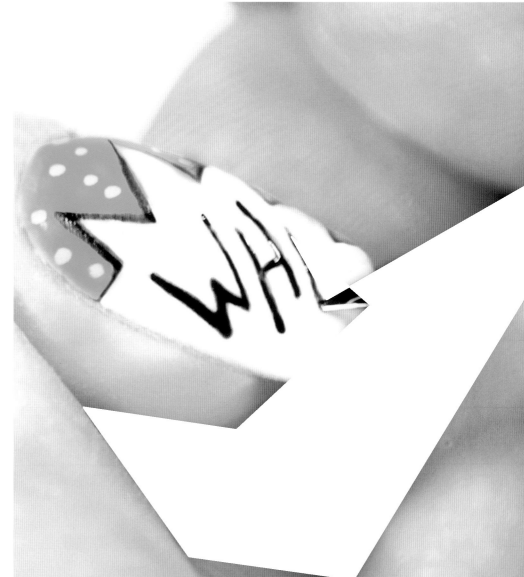

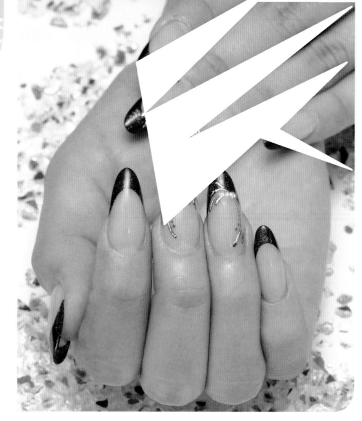

Vintage Chic

Intrinsically glamorous with a dash of sex appeal, the modern take on vintage style calls for a well-groomed finish. Classic shades of red and nude as well as natural-looking manicures take precedence to channel the feminine styles of the 1920s, and nails are largely simple in design. A half-moon manicure with a coloured moon shape at the base of the nail pays homage to the iconic style of the early 1900s, and a key shade can be chosen to complement a specific item of clothing and add the finishing touch to an ensemble.

Heading into the 1950s, shades of scarlet remained dominant to match lipstick, but experimentation began to occur. Take elements from polka dot fabrics and period films to translate styles from the era onto nails, but keep the colour and design simple, allowing clothing to be the main focus. Nails should complement fabrics by either replicating a simple pattern or matching the key shade. If you are using more than one shade, opt for different sides of the colour spectrum; avoid using colours together that have similar base hues, such as oranges, reds and pinks, and instead consider using a bold colour with a light shade to add contrast and impact.

Above left *Elegant almond-shaped nails by Eva Darabos, with a black French-style tip and pretty silver detailing.*

Left *A modern twist on a vintage look – stiletto-shaped nail extensions with a French-style tip in red with white dots and sculpted bow embellishments, by Paulina Zdrada.*

Opposite top right *Scarlet square nails with glitter and freehand detail on the ring finger by Eva Darabos.*

Opposite top left *Angular nail enhancements with multi-coloured square detailing at the tip by Gemma Lambert.*

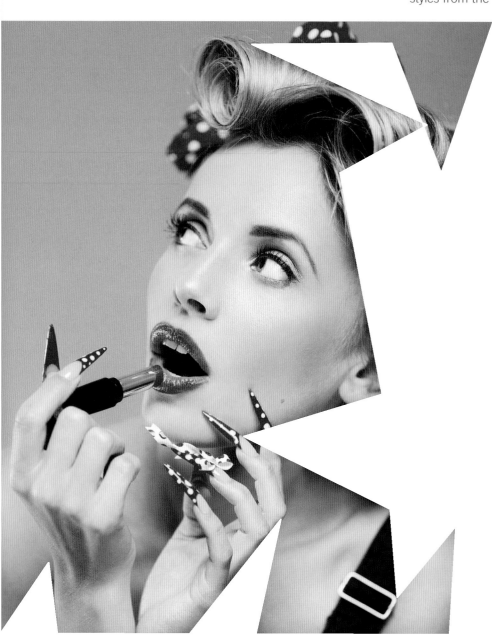

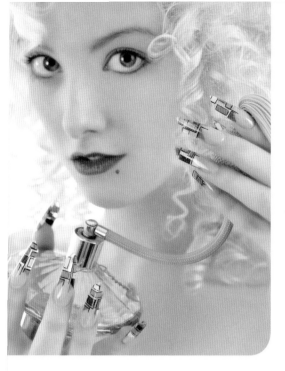
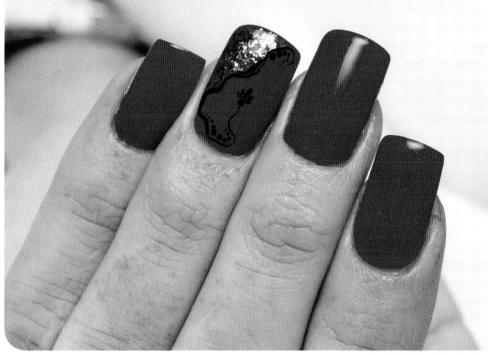

PROJECT: DOTTY ABOUT YOU by Sam Biddle

You will need

1 Base coat

2 Two nail shades

3 White nail shade for dots

4 Dotting tool or toothpick

5 Top coat

Pretty and eye-catching, a dotted design for nails is simple and speedy to achieve while offering an element of 1950s style. Sam Biddle shows how to create it in just three steps.

1 After an application of base coat, paint one of your chosen nail shades in two thin coats on eight nails, leaving the ring-finger nails bare. Next, paint the ring-finger nails in a contrasting shade in two thin layers.

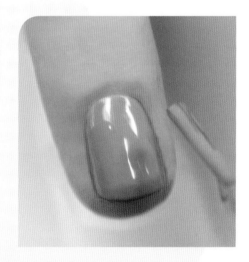

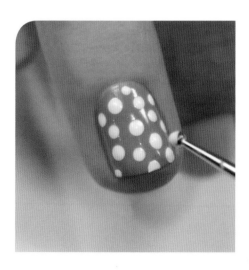

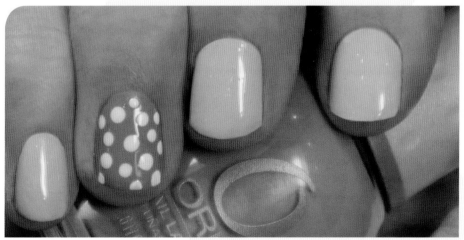

2 Dip the end of a dotting tool or small toothpick into white polish and randomly dot the ring-finger nails.

3 Allow to dry fully and apply a top coat, remembering to seal the free edge of the nail to prevent premature chipping.

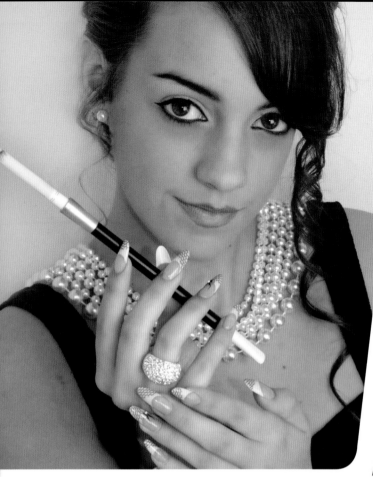

Period Designs

Iconic decades or even longer periods of time can prove inspirational when it comes to selecting colour and imagining design. The general tastes of that era, whether classic and elegant or bright and funky, can dictate length, shape and the shades used. You may wish to use your nail style to pay homage to a movement, revolution or general period in history that interests you; look to textbooks or the internet to research the iconic designs and patterns representative of these eras to aid your nail style.

Left *An Audrey Hepburn-inspired look by Gemma Lambert, with extended almond-shaped nails and subtle lace detail.*

Below *Cameo-inspired pink and black stiletto-shaped nails by Michelle Sproat.*

Opposite *A 1960s-style pink and purple pattern, painted freehand by Sophie Harris-Greenslade.*

Below *Egyptian-themed nails in an almond shape, featuring freehand designs and details by Fleury Rose.*

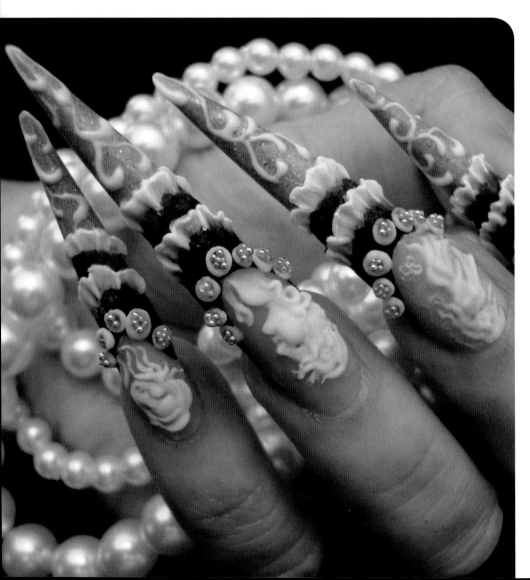

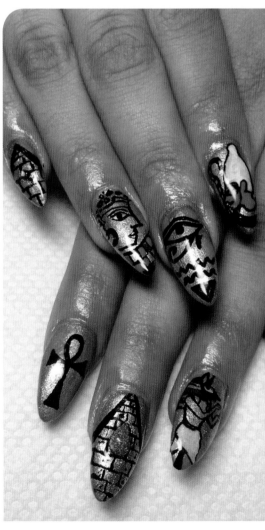

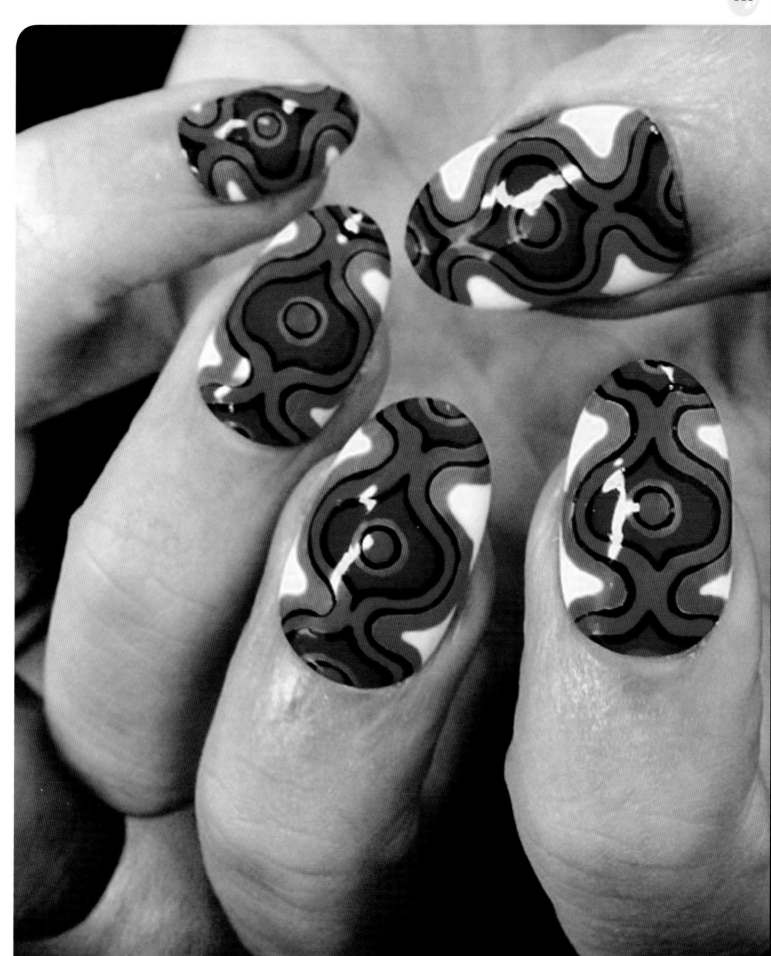

Mad for Monochrome

The combination of black and white is always striking, and using it in nail designs makes the nails eye-catching while still suitable for complementing the majority of outfits. The mod subculture of the 1960s popularized black and white clothing, paired with false eyelashes, heavy eyeliner and pale or white lipstick. Its revival is apparent in the modern fashion world, with plain white or black nails offering a chic appearance while being quick to achieve.

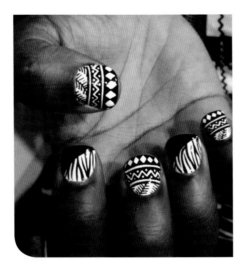

Left *Tribal-style prints meet monochrome shades in a design by Sophie Harris-Greenslade.*

Below *Almond-shaped nails with a monochrome design and a touch of mint green, by Ami Vega*

Below left *A monochrome nail design on almond-shaped nails by Sophie Harris-Greenslade, incorporating the 'halo' manicure design and a half-moon effect on feature nails.*

Opposite top left *A striking kaleidoscope-inspired design by Sophie Harris-Greenslade, using polish shades in black, white and shades of grey.*

Opposite top right *Intricate hand-painted nail art in black and white by Sophie Harris-Greenslade, created on square nails.*

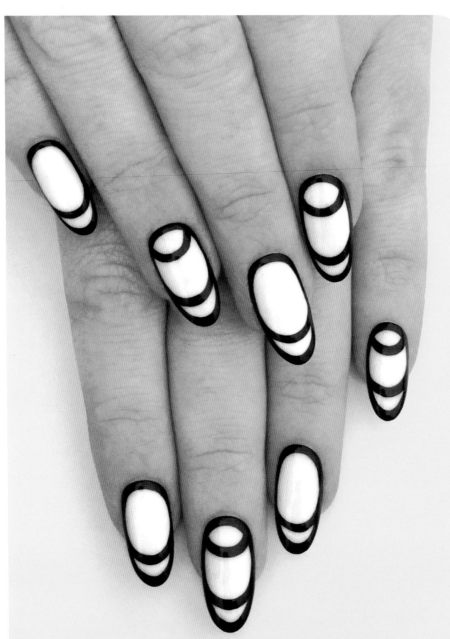

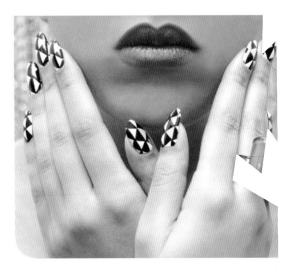

Right *A combination of monochrome designs for a random, eye-catching nail effect by Sophie Harris-Greenslade.*

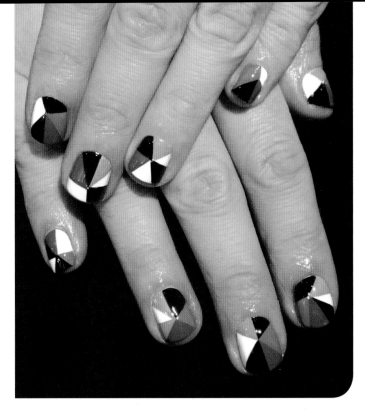

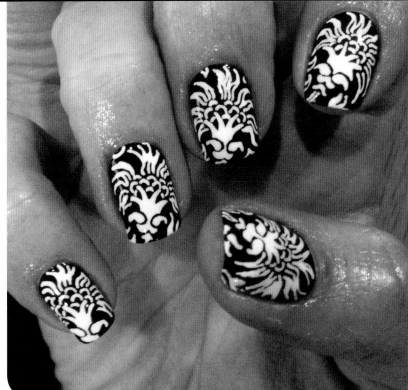

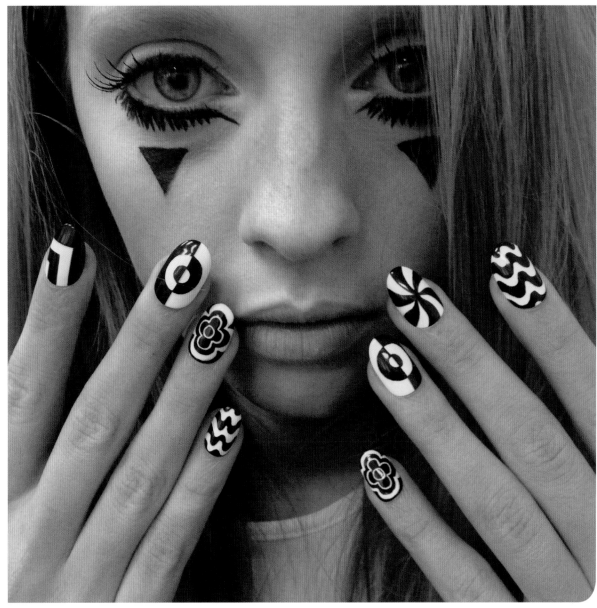

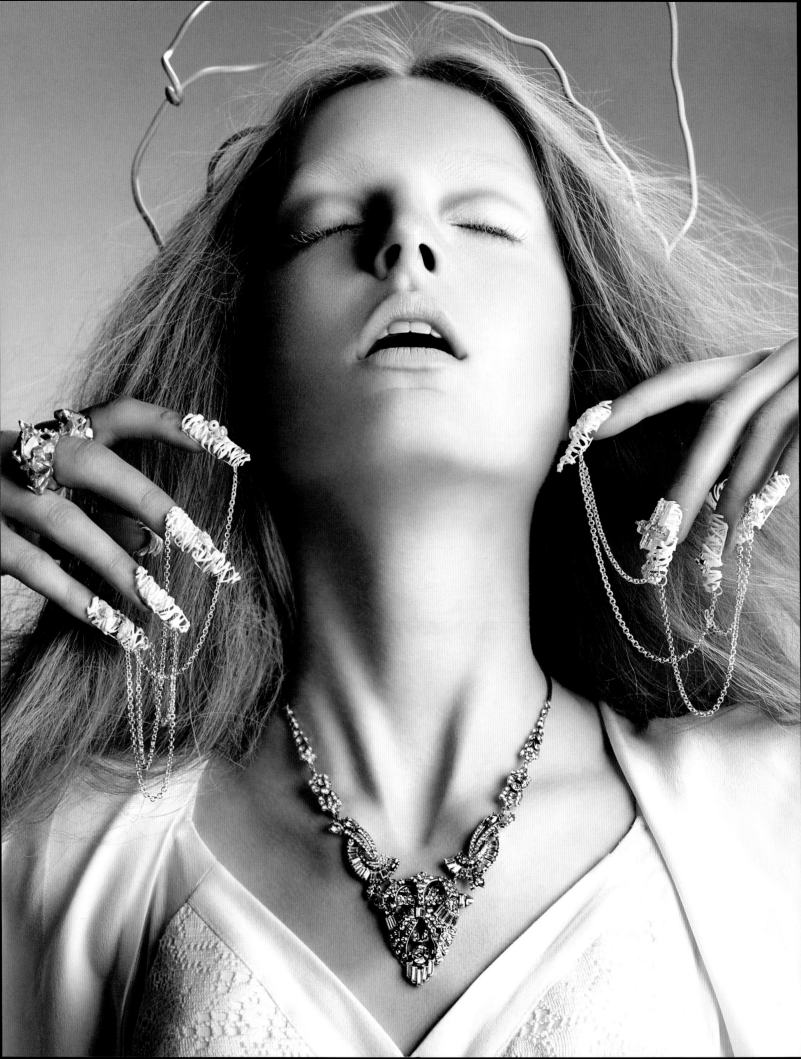

CHAPTER EIGHT

FROM THE IMAGINATION

The imagination can be the greatest tool in conjuring up unique nail styles that are personal to the creator. Leading technicians have often executed designs based on stories, visualizing the colours and aesthetics of the characters and translating them into artistry with professional products. Imaginative designs mean something different to every individual; each constructs an interpretation of a story, film, location, event, character or even dream from his or her own view, coloured by particular experiences.

Pictures formed in the mind can be random in content, colourful or black or white – and the beauty of nail products is the ease with which they allow these mental images to be transformed into visual works. Creative individuals can take elements of their imaginative ideas to create art that's different on each nail, in varying colours, and the shape of the nail can help to project the theme or idea.

Left *An ethereal 3D white nail design with chains by Sam Biddle. The nails are long to exude femininity.*

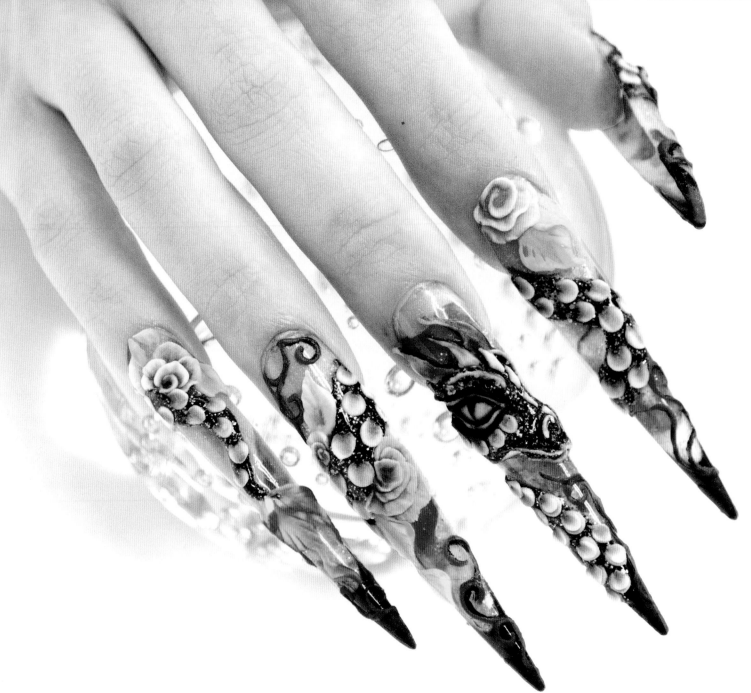

Above *An intricate nail design on stiletto-shaped, enhanced nails created with L&P acrylic products, featuring a sculpted dragon and flowers.*

Opposite top *Nails with a bridal feel, featuring nail tips of an unusual shape, hand-painted designs and a variety of sparkling decals and beads.*

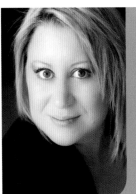

TECHNICIAN PROFILE
Viv Simmonds, Australia

With more than 20 years' experience in the nail industry, Viv Simmonds has achieved international status through her accomplishments, which include winning in excess of 50 nail competition trophies and taking the title of Australian Champion for five consecutive years.

Viv has judged nail competitions internationally and created front covers for a number of leading nail magazines, as well as appearing on television and in consumer magazines. She was listed in the Who's Who of Australian Women in 2010 and 2011 and has her own Australian Nail Team, the members of which she has trained and watched develop into multi-award-winning nail artists. Viv co-ordinates the annual Global Nail Design Awards and travels all over the world to conduct unique training events in advanced nail technology and design.

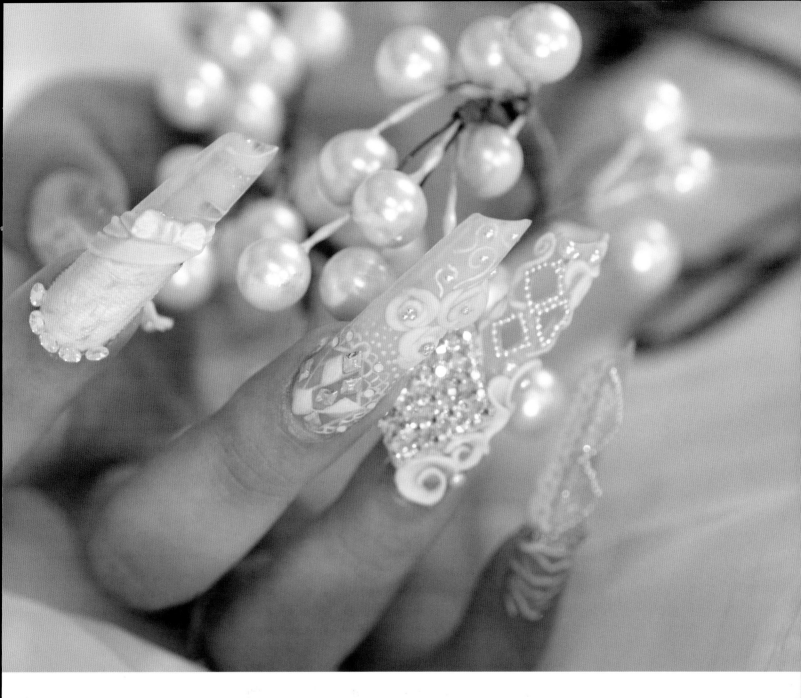

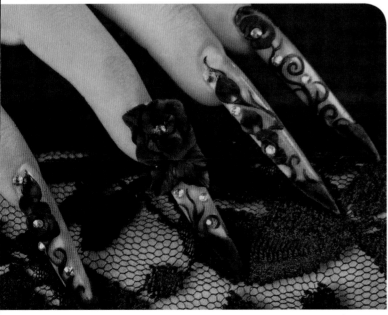

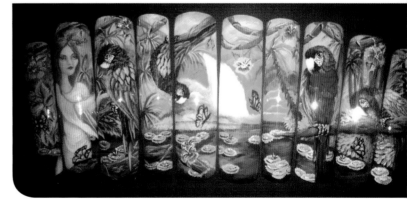

Left *Gothic-style stiletto-shaped nails with a touch of feminine pink, featuring sculpted black flowers and diamanté details.*

Above *A hand-painted, colourful design with a jungle theme on nail tips.*

Image Gallery

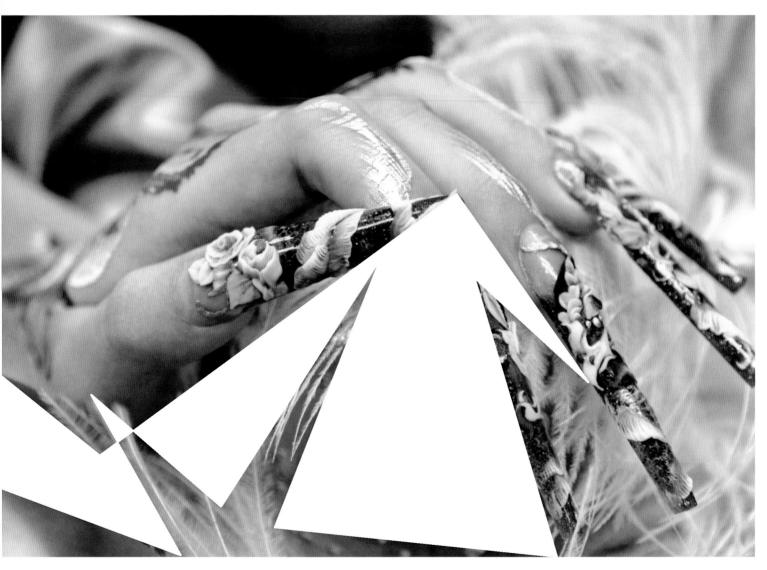

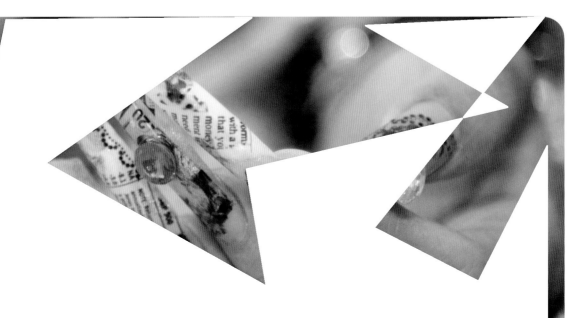

Above *Bright flowers and feathers feature in a stiletto-shaped nail design by Catherine Wong.*

Left *Sculpted enhancements with encapsulated mystical detailing and embellishments by Catherine Wong.*

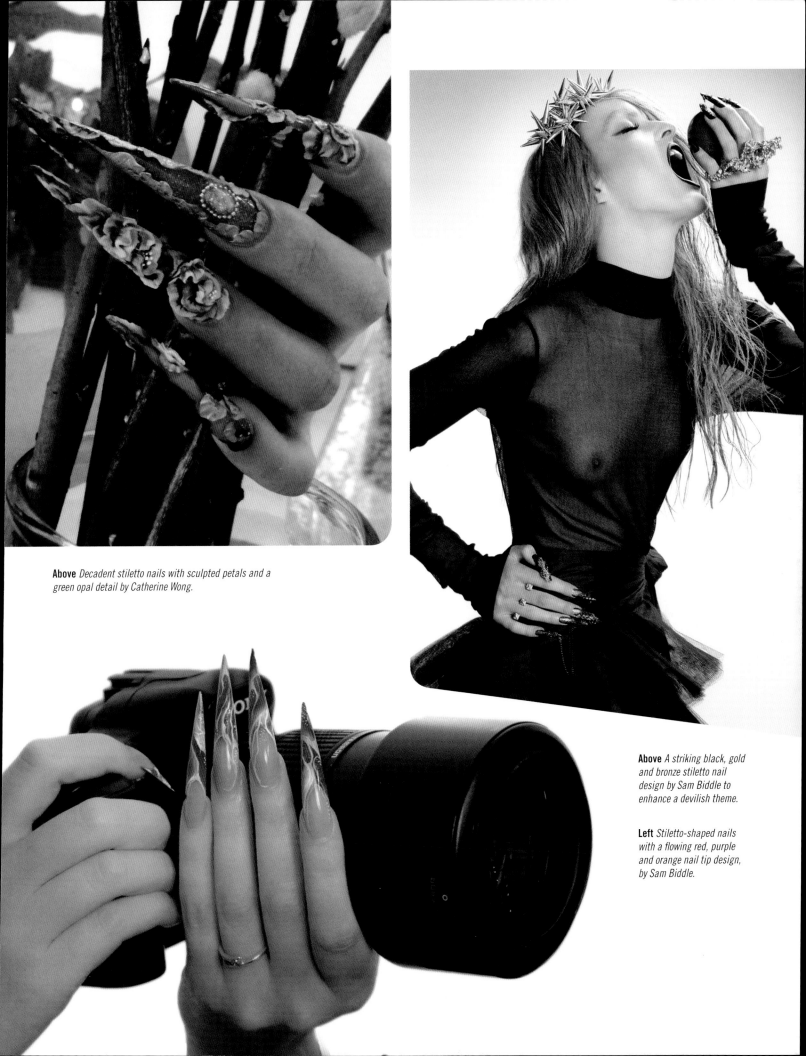

Above *Decadent stiletto nails with sculpted petals and a green opal detail by Catherine Wong.*

Above *A striking black, gold and bronze stiletto nail design by Sam Biddle to enhance a devilish theme.*

Left *Stiletto-shaped nails with a flowing red, purple and orange nail tip design, by Sam Biddle.*

PROJECT: KALEIDOSCOPIC NAILS by Sophie Harris-Greenslade

You will need

1 Base coat

2 White nail polish

3 Nail art pens in pale pink, neon pink, silver glitter, blue, green, yellow and orange (alternatively, you can use nail polish and a thin brush)

4 Top coat

For this project, experiment with a variety of colours to create an interesting and eye-catching design. Sophie Harris-Greenslade shows how in 10 steps.

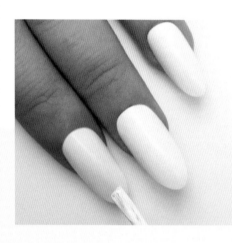

1 After applying a base coat, paint two coats of white nail polish on all 10 nails.

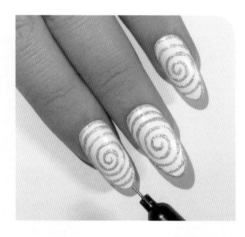

2 Using a silver glitter nail art pen (or a brush dipped in silver glitter polish), draw a swirl from the middle of each nail all the way out to the edge. Draw an outline all the way around each nail.

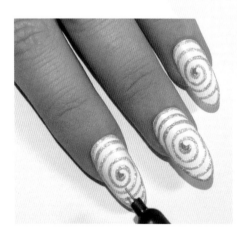

3 With a neon pink nail art pen, draw a small crescent-moon shape at the beginning of the swirl in the middle of the nail.

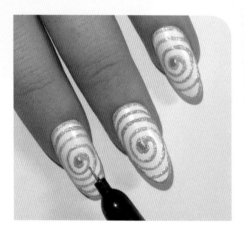

4 Leaving a small line of white, paint on another section using a green nail art pen. Each colour section needs to curve around the swirl in a crescent shape.

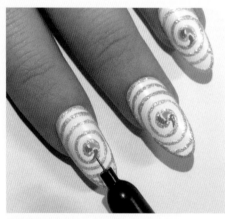

5 Leaving a small line of white, paint on a blue crescent section.

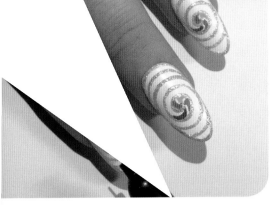

6 Repeat with orange, leaving a small line of white in between.

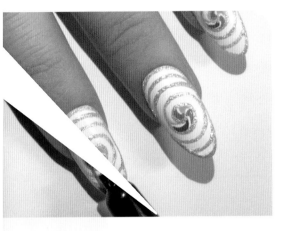

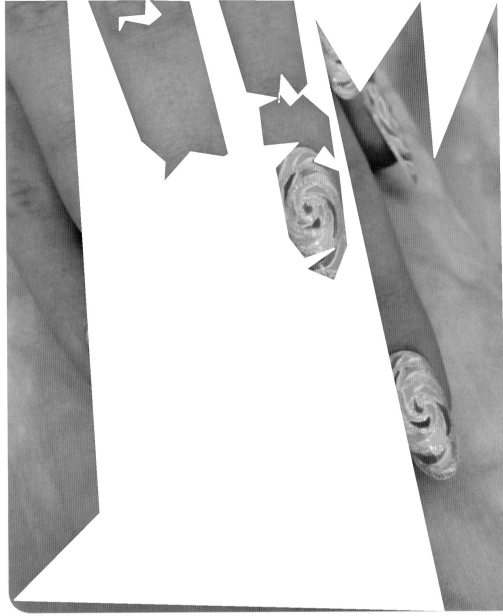

7 Repeat with yellow, following the silver glitter outline.

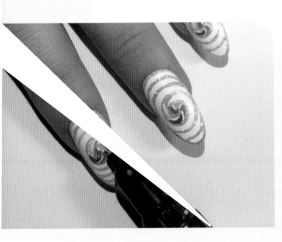

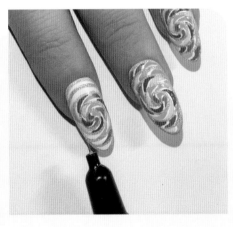

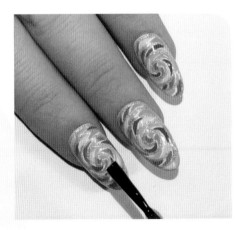

8 Continue to follow the outline on each nail and use a pale pink pen to create the next curved shapes.

9 Repeat the whole way around the swirl until you have filled the whole nail. You can use alternative colours if desired.

10 Finish the nails by applying a top coat.

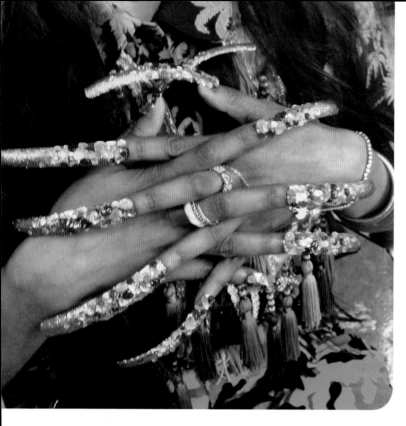

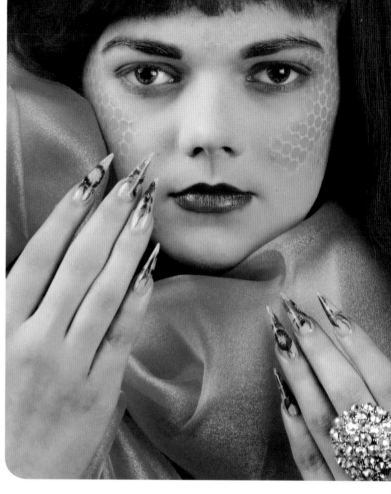

Image Gallery

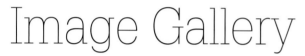

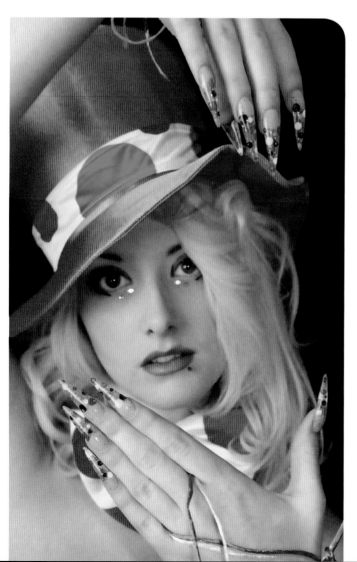

Above left *Exaggerated gold glitter nails with multi-coloured diamanté embellishments for singer M.I.A by Sophie Harris-Greenslade.*

Above *Stiletto-shaped enhancements with hand-painted floral designs by Gemma Lambert.*

Left *Clear stiletto enhancements with colour-popping dotted details by Gemma Lambert.*

Right *Playful multi-coloured patchwork nail art on extended nails by Gemma Lambert.*

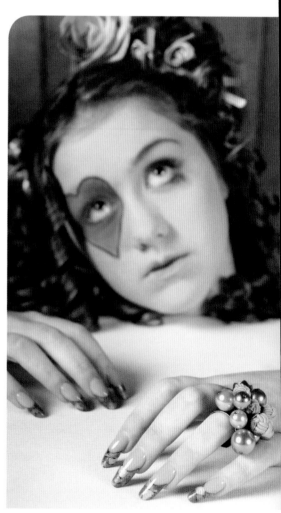

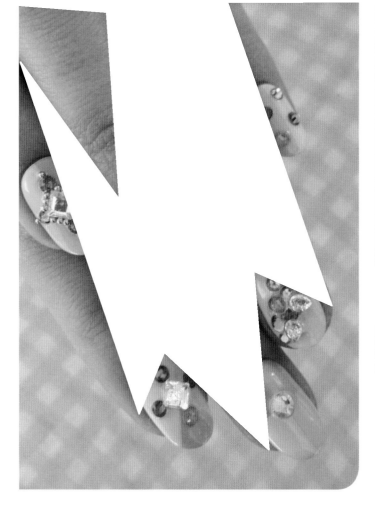

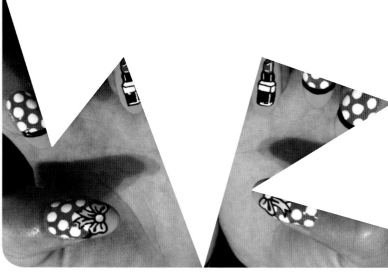

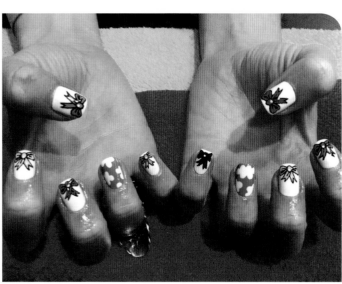

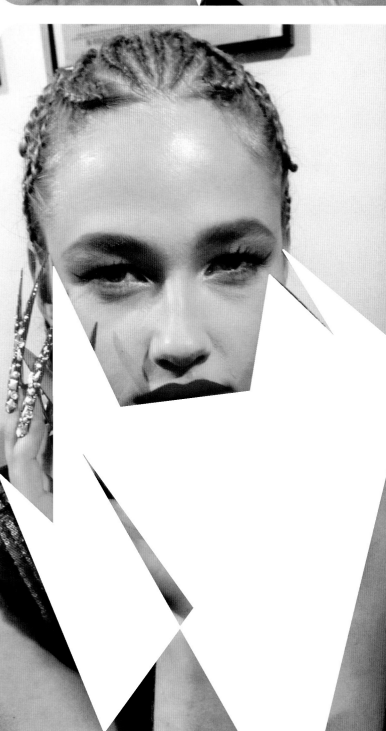

Top left *Nails with a pastel geometric design and multi-coloured stone embellishments by Sophie Harris-Greenslade.*

Top right *Playful polka-dot nails with hand-painted lipstick details on the ring fingers and bows on the thumbs by Sophie Harris-Greenslade.*

Above *Blue skies and hand-painted bright bows created on natural nails by Sophie Harris-Greenslade.*

Right *Hot pink stiletto nails with gold studs and rectangular rhinestones by Sophie Harris-Greenslade.*

Picture credits & acknowledgements

Front cover ©
Title page ©
Half title page ©
4L, 6, 7T © Sophie Harris-Greenslade; **4C, 7BR** © Samantha Morales; **7BL** © Charlotte Green; **8, 9** © Nubar UK.

Chapter 1
10, 16–17 © Charlotte Green; **12BL** © Nicola Jackson; **13** © Fleury Rose; **14** © Christina Wong; **12TL, 15TL, 15TR, 15C, 20BR, 21B** © Sam Biddle; **15BL, 15BR, 20TL, 20TR, 20C, 20BL** © Eva Darabos; **18–19** © Michelle Sproat; **21TR** © Megumi Mizuno.

Chapter 2
22, 28BR, 29, 30-31 © Samantha Morales; **24–25** © Astrowifey; **26TL, 26TR, 26B, 32** © Fleury Rose; **27TL, 27BL** © House of Holland for Elegant Touch; **27R, 33BL** © Sam Biddle; **28** © Ami Vega; **33T** © Sophie Harris Greenslade; **33BR** © Megumi Mizuno; **34–35** © Vu Nguyen.

Chapter 3
38B, 39CL, 48BL, 49BL, 54BR; 55TL, 55BR © Megumi Mizuno; **39TL, 48BL, 48BR** © Eva Darabos; **39TR, 49TL, 49TR, 50–51, 55TR, 55CR** © Fleury Rose; **39CR, 39BL, 49BR** © Sam Biddle; **39BR, 40–47 54BL** © Sophie Harris-Greenslade; **52–53** © Christina Wong; **54T** © Ami Vega; **55BL** © Helena Tepley; **56–57** © Raquel Olivo, Hand Model – Ashley Frey, Stylist – Arturo D. Chavez.

Chapter 4
58, 60BR, 61T, 61BR, 63T, 63BL, 66TL, 66TR, 66BL, 66C, 68-71, 74 © CND (Creative Nail Design Inc.); **60T, 61BL, 62, 63BC, 63BR, 64–65, 75BR** © Andrea Benedetti; **67TL, 67TR, 67BR** © Sophie Harris-Greenslade; **67BL** © Astrowifey; **72-73** © Amanda Fontanarrosa; **75T, 75BL** © Fleury Rose; **76–79** © House of Holland for Elegant Touch; **80–81** © Sam Biddle

Chapter 5
82, 84–85, 88–89, 90CL, 90BL © Eva Darabos; **86T** © Michelle Sproat; **86B** © Megumi Mizuno; **87TL, 87TR, 91TR, 91BL** © Sophie Harris-Greenslade; **87B, 91BR** © Sam Biddle; **90TL** © Christina Wong; **91TL** © Fleury Rose.

Chapter 6
92, 94B, 95L © Charlotte Green; **94L, 95R** © Nicola Jackson; **97TR** © Nicola Jackson; **104–105** © Gemma Lambert; **96TL** © Christina Wong; **96BL, 96BR, 98BR, 100TL, 100TR, 100BL, 101T, 102–103** © Sam Biddle; **97BR, 98TL, 98BL** © Eva Darabos; **97BL** © Susan Renee Photography and Sammy Grant; **99** © Megumi Mizuno; **100BR, 101BL, 101BR** © Sophie Harris-Greenslade.

Stockists

Be Creative **www.sambiddle.co.uk**

CND **www.cnd.com / www.sweetsquared.com**

Elegant Touch **www.eleganttouch.com**

Nubar **www.bynubar.com / www.palmsextra.com**

Orly **www.orlybeauty.com / www.orlybeauty.co.uk**

Chapter 7

106 © Raquel Olivo; **108–109, 111C, 111BL, 111BR** © Sam Biddle; **110BL** © Paulina Zdrada; **110TL 111TR** © Eva Darabos; **111TL** © Nicola Jackson; **112TL** © Gary Lewis; **112BL** © Michelle Sproat; **112BR** © Fleury Rose; **113, 114, 115TR, 115TL** © Sophie Harris-Greenslade; **115B** © Samantha Morales.

Chapter 8

116 © Jenny Brough; **121TR, 121B** © Sam Biddle; **118–119** © Viv Simmonds; **120 120, 121TL** © Christina Wong; **122–123, 124TL, 125** © Sophie Harris-Greenslade; **124TR, 124BR** © Charlotte Green; **124BL** © Gary Lewis.

Thanks to:

Brian Biggs, Monica Biggs, Alex Fox, Scott Derbyshire, Janine Derbyshire, Kayleigh Baker, Lizzie Benton, Fleury Rose, Christina Loglisci, Michelle Sproat, Sam Biddle, Gemma Lambert, Lucy Dartford PR, Eva Darabos, Megumi Mizuno, Ami Vega, Ashley Crowe, Sophie Harris-Greenslade, Vu Nguyen, Beth Fricke, Raquel Olivo, Catherine Wong, Christina Wong, Viv Simmonds, Samantha Sweet, Katie Gray, Ashleigh Hesp, Jan Arnold, Michael van der Ham, Antonio Sacripante, Sara Wang, Amanda Fontanarrosa, The Communications Store.